Metaphors of Coronavirus

Jonathan Charteris-Black

Metaphors of Coronavirus

Invisible Enemy or Zombie Apocalypse?

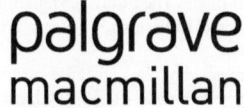

Jonathan Charteris-Black
Arts, Creative Industries, and Education
University of the West of England
Bristol, UK

ISBN 978-3-030-85105-7   ISBN 978-3-030-85106-4   (eBook)
https://doi.org/10.1007/978-3-030-85106-4

This Palgrave Macmillan imprint is published by the registered company Springer Nature Switzerland AG.
The registered company address is: Gewerbestrasse 11, 6330 Cham, Switzerland

This book is dedicated to my mother, Pauline, who did not survive the pandemic, and all those who suffered bereavement during the time of Coronavirus.

Acknowledgements

Writing this book has been a solitary exercise as, along with many other writers, researchers and other 'non-key' human beings, I have been largely restricted to home. This has made reliance on various online sources essential for its completion; in particular, I would like to acknowledge and thank all the journalists and their newspapers (accessed via the Nexis database), contributors to social media and other public platforms who have written about the pandemic, and respondents to my online survey. Without all of these the book would have been *virtually* impossible to research.

I would also like to thank my students Jessica Freathy and Megan Crouch who assisted with devising, distributing and collating the results of the Coronavirus Metaphor Survey and with the analysis of the "We are the virus" meme. I would like to thank Professor Clive Seale, for help with statistical testing and Chris Beckett for advice on the manuscript. I would also like to thank my kind partner Clare Gardner-Medwin for always trying to say something encouraging about chapter drafts.

Finally, I would like to thank all those who take an interest in reading and thinking about metaphor and provide me with the motivation to write about it.

Contents

List of Figures

List of Figures

List of Tables

1

Moral Frames and Coronavirus

Introduction

From the beginning of the year 2020 the black swan was rapidly approaching. For years western scientists had warned about the possibility of a serious pandemic, but biased thinking led politicians to believe that any novel, viral infection would probably be restricted to South-East Asia, China or Africa. After all, this had been the case with previous infectious pathogens such as Ebola, bird flu, SARS or swine flu and so, it was assumed, it would continue to be the case with future pathogens. In spite of endless global movements of products and of people, in spite of deforestation and disruption of animal habitats few believed that the transmission of a virus from animals to humans could threaten *all* of humanity. But then nobody believed that in spite of the theoretical possibility of a black swan, there actually was one, until, that is, one was discovered. With the benefit of hindsight, the reality of a global pandemic was a question of when, not if, and the black swan spread its wings across the globe.[1]

The 2020 pandemic disrupted our sense of normality, and by 'our' I mean, for the first time in history, nearly everyone. Just as trade had

© The Author(s), under exclusive license to Springer Nature Switzerland AG 2021
J. Charteris-Black, *Metaphors of Coronavirus*,
https://doi.org/10.1007/978-3-030-85106-4_1

flowed with increasing velocity under the mediating influence of technology, and global wealth had risen year on year, with gaping divergences in its distribution both between nations and among peoples within those nations, so had the assumption of human invulnerability. We might be playing Russian roulette with the climate, but it was a gamble that was worth taking for the advances that technology could bring in terms of human wealth and happiness. Ultimately, reason was in control and threats could be met with a swift, scientific response—until, that is, Covid-19. Suddenly, there was an inversion of the normal order: the more people lived in proximity with strangers in the advanced urban economies, the more they were exposed to the virus. Dispersed people living in remote places, on hillsides or on the margin of forests were now safer than populations teeming in infected cities, inside city apartments or crowded multi-generational houses. The world was turned upside down: the black swan disrupted every expectation.

There was disruption too, as political systems became inverted: those that had been liberal democracies previously now imposed the type of restrictions on personal liberty that is normally associated with authoritarian states, while some previously authoritarian states now opposed placing too rigid restrictions on individual rights. The definition of liberty changed: was freedom wearing a mask and staying in, or not wearing one and going out? Time also inverted and went back to the 1950s, when overseas travel was beyond the dreams of most, when people stayed within their localities and life was centred on the home. It was back to the simple pleasures of darning, and baking, gardening and watching the sunset. Time was something that we had assumed was forwards into a technologically driven future. Now online meetings and Webinars, online birthday parties and dinners bore a faded sepia look, like people crowding around a wireless to listen to the latest news from the frontline, and the landscape took on a slightly surreal glow. Many spoke of a disrupted sense of time: was it passing slowly or rapidly? As diaries emptied, the days took on a slower rhythm based around shopping for food, cooking and exercise and people wrote journals instead. There were household tasks and catching up with the emails, followed by perusal of the latest Netflix offerings. I have even found a diary entry: 'polish the furniture', and this regularity made us more aware of time passing. But then a month or two or three would pass so that time appeared to be accelerating. There was less to *talk about*, but more to *say*: nobody could really be doing much because nothing much was 'allowed', but they could be thinking and reflecting more deeply about what, if anything, it all meant.

Usually, we imagine children as being the most vulnerable to viruses, and yet coronavirus again upset the barrel: children's immune systems seemed to be barely affected while older people were most at risk. Normally the desire to protect others is most intensely evoked in relation to children: it is stressful to see any child suffer and terrible to see our own children in pain. The concept of cuteness triggers an emotional response of care and protection so that we want to comfort by cuddling. Yet this virus affected those who were already most physically distant—the elderly whose clear eyes had been replaced with rheumy ones and whose wrinkled skin replaced soft skin, and whose tired old limbs replaced bouncy zestful bodies. Often there are physical barriers to bodily proximity with the elderly, surrounded by frames, commodes, wheelchairs and a whole apparatus of mobility making it hazardous to approach them. Yet, it was these already distanced people who were suddenly coerced into isolation, who had to be contacted remotely or viewed through screens like aging carp in a fishpond. Enforcing the morality of care often entailed, inadvertently, enforcing a psychology of loneliness and estrangement. It was not only coronavirus that killed, but it was also the regime of separation that accompanied it.

All my mother had talked about since August 2020 was the prospect of Christmas together with family in her own home; would we have turkey or maybe a goose this year? Which bedrooms would we use? Would the girls be able to come? Would we buy a new tree or dig up the one in the garden? In the absence of other things to look forward to everything became focused on Christmas. So it came as shock when just 5 days before Christmas, with the food already bought and plans already laid, we were instructed by the Prime Minister not to travel and I was obliged to stay in a city 100 miles away from her and she would now be spending it alone. On Christmas morning she fell and broke her leg. She had an operation two days later but did not recover from the anesthetic. Though she was not as lonely as many 90-year-olds, the decision to cancel Christmas was devastating for her and presented me with a moral dilemma: should I break the rules and travel anyway, or should I leave her to Christmas alone? I was surely not alone in having to face such moral dilemmas. My mother may have died anyway irrespective of the pandemic, but the uncertainty surrounding it surely affected her zest for life. When I asked her how it compared with the Second World War, she said the pandemic was far worse because the war had brought people closer together whereas the pandemic forced them further apart.

Life and death risks are confusing: think of Orpheus and Eurydice. Orpheus was in love with a wood nymph called Eurydice, but she died after being bitten by a snake and departed to Hades' realm: The Underworld. Unable to give up the possibility of seeing her again, Orpheus stuck a deal with Hades that Eurydice could return to the world of the living as long as he, Orpheus, waited until she got into daylight before looking back. Determined to follow the rules, just as he was approaching the gates out of the Underworld, Orpheus could not stop himself from turning around just to check that she was there, but he had broken the rules and Eurydice was forced back into the Underworld for eternity.

Consider for a moment three things about this allegory: why had this condition been set? Why could Orpheus not stop himself? And thirdly what does this tell us about moral decision-making in the pandemic? There would have been no point in setting the condition about not looking back unless Hades knew that it could be broken. Second, many of our actions are instinctive and beyond our rational control: Orpheus just could not stop himself from looking back to check if she was there because his love for Eurydice was so great. We sometimes do things that we know that we shouldn't because our actions are beyond the control of our conscious thought. Third: how is this myth relevant to the pandemic? Well, it tells us that many of the Lockdown rules were set precisely because they could, or might, be broken. I suspect at least half the population at some point broke one or more of the rules, sometimes unconsciously, sometimes knowingly and sometimes with willful ignorance. And when they did break the rules, very few of them were prepared to admit to that afterwards. Moral decision making during the pandemic can be understood with reference to the allegories and metaphors that form the moral frames for these choices. The aim of this book is to examine the metaphors and allegories of the Coronavirus pandemic that give insight into the moral frames of our decision making.

Metaphor allows us to frame a moral dilemma in such a way that explains the psychological basis for the decisions we take. If we thought of the NHS staff who cared for our loved ones as 'guardian angels', we would more readily agree to their hospitalization. If we were 'fighting a war' against a virus, we might evoke appropriate emotions, and so it became acceptable to speak of activating society's resources—people, knowledge, kindness—as a 'mobilization'. Scarborough football club has a motto with a Latin origin which translates as 'No battle, no victory'. This does not mean that every time they play, they are encouraged to kick the legs off the opposition, it is intended to motivate through a commitment to winning and to argue that the attainment of success requires the maximum effort of every player. As Daniel Defoe wrote when describing the Great Plague of London in 1665: "Certainly the circumstances of the deliverance, as well as *the terrible enemy we were delivered from*, called upon the whole nation for it".[2] By framing the plague as 'the terrible enemy' Defoe was not commenting on an intention to harm people but on an appropriate emotional state for undertaking the necessary actions to protect them, so the moral foundation of Care and Harm justifies the choice of metaphor and provides insight into its moral basis. Going a stage further: if a virus is referred to as a 'zombie', because we know that zombies threaten humans, we might find a higher level of commitment towards whatever actions eliminate zombies than if we referred to it just as a virus. It is easier to imagine killing a zombie as compared with suppressing an infection and so if a pandemic is framed as a 'zombie apocalypse', then we might already know some of the strategies for staying alive. Metaphors contribute to the moral framing of a situation in such a way that we become biased towards one form of action over another, and they provide insight into the moral framing of our actions.

Moral Frames and the Pandemic

In this chapter I consider how responses to coronavirus were construed in terms of moral decision-making: decisions such as whether to visit an elderly relative, or when and how to wear a mask, whether or not to stay in the city, or—should the option be available—flee to a second home in the countryside. The chapter will be structured using the framework of Jonathan Haidt in his book *The Righteous Mind* where he argues for a 'social intuitionist model of moral judgment' in which there is no dichotomy between emotion and cognition. He proposes that emotional intuitions are themselves a form of cognition, so taking a contemporary example, continually hearing the sound of ambulance sirens is likely to trigger those parts of the brain that both arouse attention and create emotional alarm. There is no fundamental split between having our attention alerted as to an emergency vehicle and the types of emotions, fears etc. that derive from our experience of emergencies that it brings to mind.

To explain the power of moral intuitions he employs a metaphor that is part of a fable: the elephant and the rider. The 'rider' is a metaphor for the rational mind in which control derives from language-based reasoning and the 'elephant' is a metaphor for the emotions and the intuitions that accompany such reasoning. When people face a moral dilemma, Haidt claims that they rely more on the elephant than on the rider, and the rider's role is to provide some post hoc justification of a decision that is made based on an emotionally motivated moral intuition. The role of the rider is to provide an account of *why* the elephant did what it did and to justify what it wants to do next. The metaphor serves as a heuristic for a position on moral decision making that gives importance to gut instincts rather than rational reflections and seems well attuned to times when populist leaders are appealing to the instinctive emotions of 'the people'. In this book I explore the evidence from metaphor and language as to how, in the transformed world of the pandemic, journalists and politicians drew on moral frames and the nature of those moral frames on which they relied.

Care and Harm

In his Moral Foundations Theory, Haidt uses the term 'foundation' to refer to 'universal cognitive modules', since these 'cognitive modules' are now more commonly referred to as 'frames', I will use this term interchangeably with 'foundations'. The first of the six moral frames that Haidt proposes underlie people's moral intuition is Care/Harm (all the moral frames come in such pairs of opposites): this is the desire to protect others—especially vulnerable groups, such as children or the elderly, cute animals or endangered species. I recall a time when a girl I knew well sought to end a relationship with her 18-year-old boyfriend. He could not accept this decision and came to her house in the early hours of the morning after getting very drunk, threw some bricks through the bay windows of the living room and pulled off a car wing mirror and threw it through her first-floor bedroom window. It shattered the glass over her bed that was adjacent to that window. Her father was on the point of rushing out into the street to confront the source of the aggression as he felt that Harm could have come to his daughter from the broken glass in the middle of the night. But she stopped him, knowing that he had an impetuous nature and pleaded with him not to go out: he was motivated by fear of harm for her, and she showed her care for him by protecting him from making matters worse in a street brawl with a drunken young man. The law took due process and this man who had turned 18 that day was taken for a night in the police cell. Maybe he is reading this book now, so the rest remains secret.

Care and Harm provided a very salient moral foundation for Coronavirus because all the resources of society had to be directed towards care and preventing harm. Nightingale hospitals were built in various locations in the United Kingdom to ensure that some form of care would be available even if the hospitals became full. Early on during the pandemic the focus was on obtaining personal protection equipment ('PPE') for those dealing with the health needs of Covid-19 patients. Societies sought to minimize the suffering of the afflicted and to prevent infection of those who weren't. Care motivated the wearing of masks, and they became a symbol of concern to protect others whereas **not** wearing masks represented concern for the loss of the personal freedoms associated with a different moral foundation—Liberty. Opposite actions gave different priorities to different moral frames: wearing a mask placed Care above Liberty, whereas not wearing one placed Liberty above Care.

Considerations of Care and Harm were sometimes therefore in conflict with those of Liberty and Oppression. When a political leader caught the virus, it sometimes came to symbolize their incompetence in responding to the pandemic. Boris Johnson and Donald Trump contracted coronavirus having not followed guidelines on social distancing and mask-wearing. President Magufuli of Tanzania said "Coronavirus, which is a devil, cannot survive in the body of Christ… It will *burn* instantly", but in spite of his metaphors, he died after refusing to wear a mask or implementing effective measures for the control of the virus. Societies that were most successful in dealing with the pandemic were those that paid most attention to the moral foundation of Care and Harm: they pulled no punches in prioritizing Care over Liberty.

Fairness and Cheating

The second of the moral frame is Fairness and Cheating; this is grounded in altruistic feelings towards unknown others, for example insisting on people's right to benefits such as free education and free healthcare. There are expectations of reciprocal altruism: if you act well then others will act in an equally altruistic fashion towards you and your group in the future. This moral foundation derives from experience of kindness from unknown others. At the age of 18, along with many others of my generation, I hitchhiked across France and Italy and took a boat to Greece. I had a backpack and a sleeping bag and slept wherever fortune found me a bed for the night. But I had to place trust in unknown strangers: why would anyone stop to pick up a scruffy and possibly slightly rank teenager? Yet they did and I got there with no mishaps, except one driver who seemed a bit unsure of the exact location of the gearstick. In those days I regularly hitchhiked around England and Ireland as well and had lifts from people in sports cars, from a famous singer, Frankie Vaughan, and from a funeral director who explained to me how to run a successful undertaking business (a skill I could have put to good use in 2020). In Ireland it was hard to find a car that would not stop for you. On another trip to South America I met a kind and intelligent hippie on an aeroplane flying from La Paz to Lima; he had made a fortune setting up a 'hole in the wall' pizza business in Capetown; he didn't speak Spanish and I had spent the last of my money on the air ticket, so he suggested I spend a few days in Lima where I assisted by translating in restaurants and showing him around the museums and he paid the expenses. He also often bought me a gift, a leather belt with Inca designs stamped on it—there were no 'special favours'. Why did he do this? And why, subsequently, did I often stop for hitchhikers? It was because helping complete strangers brings gratification and makes you feel better about yourself too. Fairness is not something that is owned by an individual it is a social value and it is based on the moral foundation of Fairness and Cheating. In the context of hitchhiking, it is like any contract, it assumes that the driver will take the hitchhiker to the intended destination without any fee or other services, and all this is based on trust. At the broader level it is because we know that Fairness will rebound to us—somewhere, somehow, and, even if it doesn't, we have greater peace of mind from believing the possibility that it might. The unspoken assumption of altruistic behaviours is that if you were in my position, you would do the same thing for me as I am now doing for you: this is reciprocal altruism.

During the pandemic there was also an outbreak of fairness: shops and supermarkets marked lines on the pavement outside their stores at 2M intervals so customers could take their turn in a queue while maintaining physical distance. But there was cheating too by those who stockpiled essential commodities such as toilet paper flour, pasta and eggs. Their actions potentially deprived others more needy than them of the chance of obtaining these goods. Some of those who were financially affected by the pandemic because their businesses had closed, or because they had been laid off by employers had to use food banks to avoid hunger. Some hotels offered their rooms to the homeless out of considerations of fairness. Some thought rich countries were cheating by buying up all the supplies of the vaccine before poor countries could get their share. Some framed their views on Fairness and Cheating with a metaphor—*We are the Virus*—that argued that coronavirus was nature's way of punishing humanity for the environmental destruction it had inflicted. This perspective on moral reciprocity frames the virus as a form of punishment. Some religious versions of this frame have deep cultural roots in fundamentalist views of the Old Testament that God would eventually punish mankind for his disobedience. Jehovah's Witnesses saw the virus, following the floods and the locust outbreaks in Africa, as heralding the long-awaited End of Times—and the Second Coming. Some Hindus thought that this was karma. Whether secular or religious, considerations of the moral foundation of Fairness and Cheating dominated and was evident in allegories and metaphors.

While fairness and cheating is quite easy to identify in relation to panic buying and looking after those who were not able to look after themselves because of their financial circumstances, it was sometimes a more complex concept than is allowed by the social intuitionist model. This is particularly the case in relation to decisions about whether to vaccinate because they rely on interpretations as to whether the body that is being protected by vaccination is the individual's body or the body politic: the social body which concepts such as 'herd immunity' assume. Sometimes an individual who may not need a vaccine, because they are healthy and have an effective immune system, may still choose to be vaccinated because they don't want to be one of a group among whom the virus can continue to circulate. Conversely, sometimes an individual with a weak immune system who really should get a vaccine may resist getting one because as a matter of conscience they feel unable to taint the sanctity of their own body, the only one they have full control over, with something that tricks it into believing that it has been infected. The decision becomes a matter of private conscience in which the individual makes a personal decision influenced by metaphoric ideas around protection and purity.

Loyalty and Betrayal

The third moral foundation according to the social intuitionist model is Loyalty and Betrayal and concerns the evolutionary advantage conferred by tribal loyalties. In William Golding's *Lord of the Flies* a group of boys are stranded on a deserted island. Without the moral codes of adults to guide them, they split into two groups around the leaders Ralph and Jack. Their nascent moral sentiments gradually disintegrate under the pressure of fear of an imagined monster and the boys divide into tribes that become entwined in a ruthless life and death struggle for domination. The boys' fears derive from ignorance: they don't know how to start a fire other than with the glasses of a fat boy called Piggy, but this boy who is less protected by tribal loyalties becomes isolated and is hunted down and sacrificed. Evolutionary advantage comes not from knowledge but from the protection offered by membership of a stronger group.

The world suffered a similar challenge to its morality during the Covid-19 pandemic, some people responded tribally by identifying with those who shared their attitude to the level of restriction they were prepared to accept. Some did not wish to sacrifice liberty because they did not believe it was a genuine crisis: it was a 'plandemic' designed by the global technological elite to attain world domination. Others were angry with those less conscientious than themselves who ignored the rules and felt that the only moral action was to report them. There was an outbreak of accusations of treachery and betrayal. Were those who reported on neighbours for breaking Lockdown rules showing Loyalty to the larger social group or themselves betraying their neighbours?

But there were also stories of great personal sacrifice for the needs of the larger group, in the United Kingdom 100,000s of people became NHS volunteers because they wished to display loyalty to those more vulnerable than themselves. People went out of their way to show loyalty and support for their pre-existing groups who were often their families or work colleagues. Health staff, care workers, personal carers, teachers and even academics went out of their way to show solidarity with colleagues by covering for them at work if they were struck down by Covid-19 or needed to isolate. People in shared accommodation, many of them young, showed loyalty to their housemates by all staying in because one of them was vulnerable. They would not be the one to betray the household, even if not a family. I will discuss how the 'social bubble' metaphor evoked the moral foundation of Loyalty.

By contrast, other interpretations of Loyalty led to the shaming of 'out' groups, for example people with underlying morbidities. This rather unpleasant term carried with it the implication that they were somehow *responsible* for their condition. This developed into a more general criticism of, for example, obesity: since the healthy did not get ill, the unhealthy were sacrificing the liberty of the rest of us. Betrayal is always a powerful moral intuition in times of danger; those who do not observe the rules could be viewed as betraying the rest of society. Interestingly, previous tribal loyalties that had emerged over Brexit between 'Leavers' and 'Remainers' soon evaporated. The fears of chaos at the borders in the lead up to the final departure of the UK from the EU were replaced by anxieties about what was arriving from across the borders. The debate soon dissipated as it appeared that national governments were faster and more efficient in vaccine procurement and in implementing vaccination programmes. At the time of writing the United Kingdom has administered 77.37 million vaccinations and 62.87% of the population have received at least one vaccination; this compares with EU countries such as Germany 65.74 million vaccinations (50.21% of population) or France—47.71 million vaccinations (47% of population).[3] The European Commission was set up to regulate business not to do business in global vaccine markets. The President of the Commission, Ursula von der Leyen, prohibited exports of vaccine to the United Kingdom thereby engaging in what was sometimes described as 'vaccine nationalism'. There may be nothing immoral about this position, but it derives its morality from the foundation of Loyalty which argues that the health needs of your own nation, or in this case group of nations, should be considered before those of other nations, and giving away vaccine betrays your group. Loyalty and Betrayal can be, like Janus, a two-faced God: if you are loyal to one group, you risk being disloyal to another.

There are cultural variations in how Loyalty and Betrayal are interpreted. In China moral concepts were based on awareness of the interdependence of citizens and their mutual obligations, if someone became ill, the rotten apple would spoil the barrel. The role of government was to suppress individualism and place emphasis on loyalty to the group by enforcing stringent Lockdown measures. There is ancient Chinese story: the Yellow Emperor was trying to find a friend and stopped to ask the boy for directions to the village where the friend lived, and the boy gave him directions. The Emperor found the boy a source of good advice on various other topics and valuing his responses asked him if he knew the best way to govern a country. The boy, who had a background in herding horse, replied with a metaphor: *you just have to drive the wild horses out of the herd.* This reply shows that the way to protect society is to ostracize those who do not obey the laws—the traitors. The allegory of herding horses illustrates how metaphor can express moral perspectives, in this case Loyalty and Betrayal.

Authority and Subversion

The moral foundation of Authority and Subversion derives from the belief that a society requires structured hierarchies. To illustrate this consider the Royal Marsden hospital website that has a page for Nurses' roles and uniforms: Matron (blue uniforms with red piping); Sister and Charge Nurse (dark blue uniform with white dots); Senior staff nurses (blue and white striped uniforms with red piping and a red belt); Staff nurse (blue and white striped uniforms with dark blue piping and a dark blue belt); Healthcare support worker (white uniform with brown or yellow piping); Housekeeper/Ward clerk (dark blue top with white polka dots and black skirt or trousers); Research nurse (a royal blue uniform with dark blue piping); Advanced nurse practitioner (dark blue uniforms); Critical care outreach nurse (dark blue uniforms with green piping) and Clinical site practitioner (dark blue uniform with yellow piping).

These are only the nurses, and presumably there are other hierarchies for doctors and consultants. Evidently a health service is structured very clearly in terms of rank and authority on the basis of qualifications, training and years of experience etc. and attention to the health needs of patients requires a highly structured hierarchy. There is a clear line of command in hospitals so that those who do not follow the rules are reprimanded by those responsible for enforcing these rules.

In June 2016, the month of the UK's Referendum, Michael Gove, a staunch supporter of leaving the EU, famously said: "I think the people in this country have had enough of experts with organisations from acronyms saying that they know what is best and getting it consistently wrong".[4] However, with the arrival of Covid-19 governments everywhere relied on the authority of experts in molecular evolution, epidemiology, clinical science and practice, modelling infectious diseases, behavioural science, statistics, virology, microbiology, social science, social psychology, economics and other disciplines. The list was so long that in statements of policy the government justified decisions with the simple claim that they were based on 'what science has advised'. Quite swiftly appeals to the desires and wishes of the 'people' were replaced by those based on the authority of 'science' which now formed the main argument for the legitimacy of their decisions. In the face of the pandemic governments sort to gain support for their policies from the health experts from whom they derived much of their authority. The enforcers of Covid-19 policies were institutions such as the police, army and civil service that gain their legitimacy from government. The moral foundation of scientific authority is discussed in Chap. 5—Epidemiology: Science, and Metaphor.

But not all accept that Authority is morally right. A very good example of Subversion is opposition to the vaccine. Some felt that loyalty to a particular faith prevented them accepting the control of a state over their body. Others did not believe that the state was necessarily governing in their interests and therefore they did not trust government and sought to subvert its authority. It is worth recalling that the idea of objecting to government on the grounds of conscience originated in *resistance to the legal requirement to be vaccinated,* not in refusing to fight a war. In Britain the Vaccination Act of 1853 ordered compulsory vaccination for infants up to 3 months old, and the Act of 1867 extended this age requirement to 14 years, adding penalties for vaccine refusal. After considerable political action by the Anti-Vaccine movement, the Vaccination Act of 1898 removed penalties and included a "conscientious objector" clause, so that parents who did not believe in vaccination's safety or efficacy could obtain an exemption certificate. The right *not* to be vaccinated was one gained through Subversion of the authority of government in the second part of the nineteenth century: vaccine resisters saw their bodies "not as potentially contagious but as highly vulnerable to contamination and violation".[5] This outlook derived from the moral foundation of Sanctity and Degradation.

Sanctity and Degradation

The background to the coronavirus pandemic was a disruption of mankind's relationship with Nature. The increasing proximity of virus-carrying-animals to human beings caused by environmental degradation had created the conditions in which coronavirus could transfer, either directly or via an intermediary, from an animal source to a human target. The Environmentalist movement had often appealed to the idealization of the Sanctity of nature. For those who believed in this, coronavirus was a potential blessing and numerous accous of man's restored relations with nature abounded on social media. A movement grew around the hashtag #WeAreTheVirus:

> Wow…Earth is recovering
>
> -Air pollution is slowing down
> -Water pollution is clearing up
> -Natural wildlife is returning home
>
> Coronavirus is Earth's vaccine
> We're the virus[6]

The concept of the Earth as sacred was powerful and overwhelming and there were tributes everywhere to Nature. The meme "We are the virus" spread widely on social media—being retweeted 70,900 times and receiving 290,900 'likes'—and this reflected a moral disgust with humanity for not respecting the sanctity of the planet. Such viewpoints could be described as; 'Eco-fascist' since there was undeniably a streak of sanctity and disgust underlying the social intuitions of some of the environmentalist movement. I discuss their metaphors and corresponding allegories in Chap. 4.

The sanctity of nature is broadly in keeping with the social intuitionist approach to moral frames. Even the Duke of Sussex expressed these sentiments:

> Prince Harry said: "Somebody said to me at the beginning of the pandemic, it's almost as though Mother Nature has sent us to our rooms for bad behaviour, to really take a moment and think about what we've done.

It's certainly reminded me about how interconnected we all are, not just as people but through nature. We take so much from her and we rarely give a lot back…At the end of the day, nature is our life source… But you can't uplift, educate and inspire unless there is a form of action that follows."[7]

In his book *Natural*, written before the pandemic, Levinovitz argues that a faith in Nature has replaced the feelings of Sanctity that were previously attributed to a divine presence, to a God. The main argument is summarised in its sub-title: "How faith in nature's goodness leads to harmful fads, unjust laws and flawed science". He explains the limitations of making a fetish out of Nature:

When the state of nature represents purity, then every fruit of modernity becomes a potential source of pollution. Food is toxic. Cribs are abusive. Unnatural lifestyles destroy our bodies. Technology destroys our souls. This mind-set conduces to deep existential anxiety which leads to the desperate piecemeal adoption of seemingly natural practices.[8]

The 'We are the virus' meme expressed a similar tendency to sanctify 'Nature' and this was clearly expressed in Prince Harry's 'Mother Nature' metaphor. Reference to 'Mother Nature' occurred in 247 news reports in the British press in the three months from 1st March 2020 as compared with only 157 times in the same period in 2019 (an increase of 57%). In this allegory, mankind was a self-seeking, greedy, voracious species that was creating the conditions for its own destruction because it was not in harmony with its environment. To some extent the pandemic appeared to be proving this to be true: the zombies were the armed forces of nature fighting back.

Shortly before the onset of the pandemic I was in a sauna at the local lido when a woman started coughing, quite loudly and repeatedly. Though I realized this was (probably) unintentional on her part, I shrunk back and felt disgusted at her behaviour. In April 2020 *MailOnline* reported that in Australia:

Under new coronavirus rules, anyone who spits or coughs on health care workers or police will be slapped with a $5000 fine.

The extreme measures were announced in response to the 'abhorrent' incidents in the last few weeks which saw nurses and police coughed or spat on during the coronavirus pandemic.

NSW Health Minister Brad Hazzard and Police Minister David Elliott said anyone found guilty of the disgusting act will cop the huge fine and possible six months in prison.[9]

An employee of London transport, Belly Mujinga, who worked at London's Victoria railway station, died two weeks after being spat at by a man who claimed he had coronavirus. The act of spitting in the presence of others is disgusting at any time, but when initiated by someone who believes themselves to be infected with Covid-19 it becomes deeply disgusting, irrespective of whether it is directed at a nurse, or anyone else.

The moral foundation of Sanctity/Degradation is based on emotions such as disgust towards dead or decaying matters or towards behaviours such as incest that challenge basic rules of morality. The feeling of disgust may have its very origin in resisting the spread of microbes, or genetic deformity and the psychologist Mark Schaller has described disgust as part of the "behavioral immune system".[10] However, a more recent study argues that findings from the human pathogen-avoidance literature shows that disgust is not useful in the context of pandemics such as Covid-19. They argue that in pandemics infected individuals are contagious before any symptoms emerge and some never develop any symptoms. Disgust in traditional societies was based on the smell of putrid food and this did not apply in relation to Covid-19.[11] However, I think that the behavioural routes through which Covid-19 is transmitted **do** evoke disgust cues. I recall feeling disgusted at the woman coughing in the sauna because one of the first described symptoms of Covid-19 was a 'dry cough'. The purpose of pathogens is endless self-replication like the infinite reflections of mirrors facing each other. Their quiet seduction of the human immune system could happen either harmlessly, without the infected even knowing, or wreak havoc in the respiratory system. Behaviours labelled 'disgusting' by the British press included stockpiling essential goods, disposing of masks in public, and the booing of the Covid vaccine by the crowd at the Australian tennis Open in February 2021. The TV host Piers Morgan furiously attacked a man who recorded himself licking a row of toiletries in a shop during the coronavirus crisis.

Sanctity and Degradation influenced the intuition of anti-vaccine supporters. The human body was degraded by injecting it with contaminants, among some Muslims there was concern that the vaccine contained pork, and in the case of Lockdown sceptics it contained a Bill Gates microchip as part of the strategy for global domination by the elite. But these beliefs based on Sanctity were themselves something of a luxury, as Kenan Malik comments:

> In countries with robust health systems, people have the dispensation to opt for natural childbirth, or alternative medicines, or reject vaccines. In much of the world in which "natural" childbirth is an imposition on women, not a choice, both maternal and infant mortality rates are staggeringly high. It is poverty that condemns so many in the global south to rely on traditional medicine or to live without vaccines…. It is the poor, whether in rich countries or in the global south, who most suffer from industrial pollution, are most imperilled by climate change and most threatened by the consequences of the coronavirus. This is not because humans are violating nature, but because societies are structured in ways that ensure that innovation and development remain the privilege of the few, while depradation and ill health are the lot of the many.[12]

Liberty and Oppression

The final moral foundation in Haidt's model, and a late addition, is Liberty/Oppression; this describes the attempts by one group to dominate another. During the Covid-19 pandemic this moral foundation was sometimes in outright conflict with other moral frames such as Care and Harm and Loyalty and Betrayal. There was an ongoing moral tension between claims for the economic freedom of the private sector and the need to prevent harm to others by allowing the spread of the virus. Then there was the question of enforced immunity by vaccination. Originally, 'immunity' referred to limits on state jurisdiction, as for example in the concept of 'diplomatic immunity' that puts limits on the scope of state authority, but in medical contexts, individuals also had the right *not* to have immunity from disease forced on them. In either case, judgements are based on notions of Liberty and Oppression.

Transcripts of the minutes leading up to George Floyd's death reveal he told officers "I can't breathe" more than 20 times, only to have his plea dismissed by Derek Chauvin, the white officer pressing his knee into Floyd's neck, who said: "It takes a heck of a lot of oxygen to talk." Floyd's dying words have become a rallying cry at demonstrations around the world amid a reckoning with systemic racism and police brutality. The chilling transcripts of body-camera video recordings that were made public provided testimony to what had happened after police apprehended Floyd on 25 May. Before he died, Floyd cried for his dead mother and his children. "Momma, I love you. Tell my kids I love them. I'm dead," he said. This united the moral frames of 'Care/Harm', 'Fairness/Cheating', 'Sanctity/Degradation' with those of Liberty/Oppression as it was not just coronavirus that affected African Americans more than it did ethnic whites, but police brutality as well! Metaphor and metonymy blended together moral intuitions about racial injustice with the pandemic because the literal act of not allowing someone to breath resulted in the same primary symptom as coronavirus. The difference being that in the one case the active agent is human, a police officer, while in the other case the virus agent does not have moral intention. The coronavirus was an invisible cloud, if you could see it, so the diagrams showed us, it would look like a sputnik, with numerous spikes emanating from a sphere that was so small that it could get inside your body and leave its own secret message, but if you wanted an allegory for it, then it was a brutal police officer crushing the breath out of George Floyd.

Yearnings for Liberty also manifested themselves against various forms of injustice with higher intensity; in my city, Bristol, rejection of the injustice of slavery, and frustration with the official channels for taking decisions about statues, led a crowd of young people to topple the statue of Edward Colston and cast it into the harbour, and it is now in a museum. Later, across the country as a whole, there was fury at the attempt to set up a soccer Super League that would permanently install a self-selecting elite of European football clubs into a new league that would not allow promotion and relegation, sealing their elevated status for eternity. Rebellions grew everywhere and the proponents of such a scheme were forced to backdown: they had infringed the Liberty of other clubs no matter how small, a right that was embedded in other competitions such as the FA Cup, which any team could enter. Then, back in Bristol, there were more than 12 demonstrations against the Police, Crime, Sentencing and Courts Bill that would make it "a criminal offence of residing in a vehicle on land without permission" that infringed on the liberty of the Gypsy, Romani and Traveller communities. The same bill warranted a sentence of up to 10 years in prison for damaging memorials. The anger against attacks on Liberty was all the greater because for so long people had already felt oppressed by coronavirus and this reflected in the rather confrontational metaphor they adopted: "Kill the Bill". Now when the agent was human it had become an allegory for Oppression. Although the virus took no prisoners, it had imprisoned society and these people now wanted a return of their freedom against apparently oppressive human agency.

A Challenge to Moral Foundations Theory: Honesty and Dishonesty

The social intuitionist model is especially well suited to the time of pandemic when daily life became a trial of minor moral decisions on issues that had not previously been matters for much reflection: whether to go out or stay at home, when and where to wear a mask, whether or not to visit elderly friends or relatives. Then there was the moral question of the possibly serious health effects of vaccination: is it right to be vaccinated to protect ourselves and others, even if this infringes our beliefs about the sanctity of the body? If we choose not to get vaccinated, should we go to public places or travel abroad? And what is the morality of so-called 'vaccine passports'—do they restrict the liberty of those who choose not to get vaccinated? Are the rights of audiences at mass events such as music festivals or sports events infringed on by those who are not vaccinated? Everywhere the pandemic brought moral dilemmas the resolution of which depended on individuals' moral intuitions. In the case of vaccine hesitancy, more than a single moral foundation applied, historically resistance to vaccination was motivated by concerns for freedom as people believed that this challenged their right to ownership of their own body;

they also supported the abolition of slavery as the two issues seemed metaphorically linked. However, they also had concerns about degradation of the sacrosanct human body, so their subversion of authority interacted with Sanctity/Degradation and Liberty/Oppression. It was probably because of the complexity of these moral concerns that governments everywhere held back from making either vaccination or vaccine passports obligatory.

Sometimes moral frames were in conflict: if one country sought to care for its citizens by obtaining limited resources such as oxygen or vaccine might that not be cheating those in other poor or middle-income countries who did not have the same access to these resources? If people in my social group avoided taking the Covid-19 vaccine because they did not trust a vaccine developed by white people, would I be betraying my loyalty to my group by getting vaccinated? If I reported someone for going out when showing symptoms of Covid-19 was I not infringing on their liberty? While ultimately moral decisions were based on intuitions about right and wrong, there was rarely a fully reasoned application of "the rules" but an act of interpretation based on gut instinct. People often blamed their confusion on 'mixed-messaging' whereas in reality their uncertainties originated in different moral frames pulling against each other.

But there is a defect in Haidt's social intuitionist theory: it overlooks Honesty and Dishonesty, which are closely related to truth telling and deception. For Haidt these are Platonic ideals and he argues that reason is not 'fit to rule' as it was designed to seek justification not truth.[13] I will argue that, in a time of pandemic, human survival depends as much on reason, the rider, as it does on the elephant of emotion. If someone asks you whether or not you have been vaccinated, surely there is an honest and a dishonest answer? Many held that the Prime Minister, Boris Johnson had lied when he claimed that Britain had met its target of 100,000 daily coronavirus tests and that ministers continued to make false claims about the numbers being tested for several more weeks.[14] Maybe this didn't matter because he was simply preserving his reputation, but in arguing against truth because our social intuitions draw on the moral frames outlined above, Haidt overlooks the fact that being honest, telling the truth, and avoiding deception, is necessary for morality because it enhances the possibility of species survival. In post-truth discourse truth had become equated with 'science' alone—and government policies always claimed to be based on 'science'. But if data are fabricated, or findings misrepresented because that tells a better narrative then this is dishonest and immoral.

Similarly, if those in positions of authority who made rules did not then follow them, then surely that was also a form of dishonesty? The British epidemiologist Neil Ferguson resigned from his position as a government advisor on the Scientific Advisory Group for Emergencies after admitting to breaking the rules on social distancing by visiting his girlfriend. His admission was honest, but his action had been dishonest. Even worse was when some in a position of authority not only broke rules but then denied having done so. This was the case when Boris Johnson's Chief Advisor Dominic Cummings appeared to break Lockdown rules by driving 264 miles from London to Durham after his wife showed symptoms of Covid-19. While in the Northeast, and on his wife's birthday, he also drove 30 miles to Barnard Castle; he claimed that this was to assess whether or not his eyesight was good enough for him to drive back to London the following day. People felt this account of his actions was at least disingenuous and probably deceptive. His later dismissal from the post of Chief Advisor suggests that dishonesty was coming to be viewed as damaging to reputation. And yet ironically the same individual relied heavily on an appeal to 'honesty' when giving evidence to Health and Social Care Committee and Science and Technology Committee on 26 May 2021 as in the following extract:

Q1016 Chair:	…but I just wanted to pick up something that you said, Mr Cummings. I think I heard you correctly in accusing the Health Secretary of having *lied*. Did I hear that correctly?
Dominic Cummings:	Yes.
Q1017 Chair:	That is obviously a serious charge. Can you provide the Committee with the evidence behind that assertion?
Dominic Cummings:	Yes. There are numerous examples. In the summer, he said that everyone who needed treatment

got the treatment that they required. He knew that that was *a lie* because he had been briefed by the chief scientific adviser and the chief medical officer himself about the first peak. We were told explicitly people did not get the treatment that they deserved. Many people were left to die in horrific circumstances.

Q1018 Chair: Is that the basis of your assertion or are there other pieces of evidence that you base that charge on?

Dominic Cummings: Yes. In mid-April, just before the Prime Minister and I were diagnosed with having covid ourselves, the Secretary of State for Health told us in the Cabinet Room, "Everything is fine on PPE. We have got it all covered," and so on. When I came back, almost the first meeting I had in the Cabinet Room was about the disaster over PPE and how we were actually completely short and hospitals all over the country were running out. The Secretary of State said in that meeting, "This is the fault of Simon Stevens; it is the fault of the Chancellor of the Exchequer. It is not my fault—they blocked approvals on all sorts of things." I said to the Cabinet Secretary, "Please investigate this and find out if it is *true*." The Cabinet Secretary came back to me and said, "It's completely *untrue*. I have lost confidence in the Secretary of State's *honesty* in these meetings."[15]

His central argument was that the Health Secretary, Matt Hancock, had repeatedly lied about the efficacy of the measures being taken to fight Covid and he often uses the phrase 'to be honest':

Q1180 Dominic Cummings: I can't really remember conversations, *to be honest*, about eat out to help out specifically.

Q1184 Chair: Okay, so you didn't oppose eat out to help out
                      because it was consistent with the strategy.
Dominic Cummings   *I honestly can't even remember* what I said about
                      eat out to help out. I didn't pay huge attention to
                      eat out to help out.

The main thrust of his rhetoric was to contrast the dishonesty of the
Health Secretary with his own honesty. The most persuasive, and, up 'til
now, among the most successful political advisors, understood the power
of appeals to moral frames based on honesty; however, on examining his
own record on this point, it was found to fall short and so his accusations
lost their sting.

Just as I was completing this book it came to light that the Health
Secretary, Matt Hancock, a married man with children, was secretly
recorded on CCTV engaged in extremely close physical intimacy, during
Lockdown, with an aide, whom he had appointed—Gina Coladangelo.
She was a former university friend and it seemed as if the affair had been
going on for some time, including the time when social distancing measures were required by government. As he was clearly breaking the rules
that he had been highly instrumental in making, he felt obliged to resign,
just before he would have been forced to do so. In this letter of resigna-
tion, he stated:

> We owe it to people who have sacrificed so much in this pandemic *to be
> honest* when we have let them down as I have done by breaching
> the guidance.

It was a lack of honesty, the very moral foundation that I propose in this
book, that led his actions to be viewed by public opinion as the epitome
of hypocrisy. *The Observer* quoted Boris Johnson's foreword to the minis-
terial code: "There must be no actual or perceived conflicts of interest.
The precious principles of public life—integrity, objectivity, accountabil-
ity, transparency, *honesty* (my italics) and leadership in the public interest—must be honoured at all times". It continued:

> Members of the public who were unable to hug loved ones before they
> died, who missed funerals and who went months without seeing newborn

grandchildren will be justified in feeling furious at a minister breaking the rules to engage in an affair. Hancock has also said that public figures in far less high-profile positions were right to resign for breaking the regulations. His hypocrisy undermines faith in the government's approach to public health during a pandemic.[16]

As I had been one of those who had been unable to see his mother before she died because of following Covid-19 rules, I also found his behaviour hypocritical and, without, I hope, sounding too self-righteous, yearn for a change in the moral foundations of public life that leads to honesty being taken more seriously.

We have seen that trust is an essential quality in several moral frames including Fairness and Cheating, Authority and Subversion, Loyalty and Betrayal as well as Honesty and Dishonesty, it therefore cuts across a range of moral judgements. Trust and reputation rely on people being candid, but they need to be so consistently if they are to be believed: candour is about behaviour and actions and how far they accord with language and discourse. Honesty is a foundation of morality but is explicitly rejected in Haidt's social intuitionist model as articulated in *The Righteous Mind*. He cites an experiment in which subjects are given verbal confirmation of how much they are paid, but when they receive the money, the cashier misreads a digit and gives them too much: only 20% correct this. But they were three times more likely to be honest when asked directly if the money was correct, with 60% saying it wasn't. He then quotes Ariely: "When given the opportunity, many honest people will cheat. In fact. Rather than finding that a few bad apples weighted the averages, we discovered that *the majority of people cheated*, and that they cheated just a little bit".[17] He argues that the 'rider' (moral reasoning) is not in charge of ethical behaviour. I don't doubt that this may sometimes be the case and I can think of several times in the past when I have not been entirely honest (and I will tell you one at the end of this book); however, in the context of the Coronavirus pandemic the risks of being dishonest are much higher: if a friend tells you they have been isolating after an overseas trip and you see them in the supermarket, the cost of their dishonesty could be other peoples' lives.

Outline of Chapters

In Chap. 2 I describe the most dominant metaphor frame during the pandemic: the 'war' frame ('frontline' and 'invisible enemy' etc.). In Chap. 3 I investigate two other very important frames: the 'fire' frame— ('sparks' or 'flare up' etc.) and what I call the 'force of nature' frame; this includes metaphors such as 'surge', 'overwhelm' and 'waves' of pandemic. When leaders spoke of 'turning the tide' against the virus they were framing coronavirus as a force of nature. Chapters 2 and 3 are based on metaphors collected from the United Kingdom's national press during a one year period from 1st March 2020 to 28th February 2021 using the theme 'Coronaviruses' on the Nexis database and on some empirical research that I undertook into the effect of different frames on people's beliefs about appropriate responses to a pandemic.

In Chap. 4 I examine the frames for articulating the existential threat to humanity posed by coronavirus and explore how the moral responses to these dangers derived from allegories taken from science fiction films and dystopic fiction. A dominant allegory for the pandemic, I suggest, is that of a zombie apocalypse. In the second part of the chapter, I discuss how moral intuitions relating to feelings of disgust about man's role in causing the pandemic manifested themselves in allegories about the Sanctity of Nature and were expressed by the "We are the virus meme" in which a metaphor expresses a viewpoint on mankind's destructive impact. Both memes, I suggest, express feelings of a loss of agency and both were somewhat fatalistic in the face of the powerful forces of nature that had been unleashed by the spread of coronavirus.

In Chap. 5 I examine metaphor frames relating to Science, I was interested in how the agency of science became a moral stick that demanded obedience. Metaphors such as 'following the science' and 'flattening the curve' were a rhetorical accompaniment to statements of government policy. I discuss 'herd immunity'—a science-based metaphor—that caused anxiety as it challenged established moral frames. Many people were confused by 'herd immunity' because it was both a technical term in epidemiology but also one that had popular connotations and carried implications when applied to the 'body politic'. Agency is always a key issue in attributing blame, and the desire to avoid blame in the future influenced many official statements on coronavirus policy but they appealed to reason rather than to Haidt's elephant of intuition.

Chapter 6 explores the cultural history of the experience of confinement in Europe. Whether it was the notion of quarantine or the 'cordon sanitaire' during periods of pandemic, there was a historical context for our experience of confinement during the 2020 pandemic—both in historical memory, in diary accounts and in cultural outputs such as cinema. Historical awareness of the plague—pest houses, doctors wearing strange bird-like masks, or Daniel Defoe's account of London during the Great Plague—influenced our frames for the coronavirus pandemic. I also explore how linguistic concepts relating to containment offer the conceptual basis for interpreting experience, whether of containment of Communism during the Cold War or views on the body as a container for the emotions.

In Chap. 7 I examine container-related metaphors that expressed moral and political viewpoints on the pandemic; these include words and phrases such as 'bubble', 'cocoon', 'bunker' and 'petri dish' all of which share container-related attributes. I explore these properties by considering the nature of the container, what is constrains, and whether the viewpoint is from outside or inside the container. At all times I am interested in how metaphors express agency and in the transitivity relationships between the entity that is contained (for example the elderly in a care home) and the entity that is imposing the containment (the government). People often felt powerless during the pandemic and it was through language that their compliance was invited, exhorted and enforced.

In Chap. 8 I consider what metonymy tells us about the moral frames of the pandemic. This is often overlooked as a trope for moral framing and by identifying key images and keywords from the British press, I consider four visual metonyms: the mask, the hazmat suit, the hearse, and the rainbow and argue that they provided mental access into moral attitudes during the pandemic. For example, in many countries, including the United Kingdom, a rainbow depicted in a window expressed the idea *E Pluribus unum* (out of many come one); this visual metonym based on the moral foundation of Care offered psychological reassurance at a time of crisis.

Finally, in Chap. 9 I consider the misinformation surrounding Covid-19 and how metaphor was used by journalists and politicians to provide a moral commentary on the advocates of 'miracle cures'—often exposing them as fake remedies. I consider how dominant metaphors such as 'magic bullet' and other metaphors related to magic such as 'magic potions' and 'magic wands' were employed by political leaders. I examine British press stories reporting on 'miracle cure' stories such as those that referred to, for example, taking hydroxychloroquine or eating garlic. In the second part I explore how the moral frames of the anti-vaccine movement take their origins in 'human as animal' metaphors and illustrate how metaphor was also employed by advocates of vaccination. In each section I suggest that metaphor was crucial in framing the debate and in articulating deeply held moral arguments drawing on both religious and humanist philosophical positions.

Notes

1. A black swan is 'Something extremely rare (or non-existent); a rarity, *rara avis*' (OED).
2. http://www.gutenberg.org/files/376/376-h/376-h.htm. Accessed 29 March 2021.
3. https://ourworldindata.org/covid-vaccinations. Accessed 29 March 2021.
4. Michael Gove, 3 June 2016.
5. Wolfe, R.M., Sharpe, L.K. Anti-vaccinationists past and present. *BMJ*. 2002d;325: 430–432.
6. Twitter 17 March 2020.
7. mirror.co.uk, 3 December 2020.
8. Levinovitz, A. (2020) *Natural: How faith in nature's goodness leads to harmful fads, unjust laws and flawed science*. Boston: Beacon Press, p. 77.
9. *MailOnline*, 17 April 2020.
10. Haidt, J. (2012) *The Righteous Mind*. London: Penguin, p. 172.

11. Ackerman, J., Tybur, J.M. & Blackwell, A.D. (2020) What Role does Pathogen Avoidance Pyschology play in Pandemics? *Trends in Cognitive Sciences*. 25: 177–186.
12. Kenan Malik in *The Observer*, 10 May 2020.
13. Haidt, J. (2012) *The Righteous Mind*. London: Penguin, p. 86.
14. A full account of such fabrications is provided in Oborne, P. (2012) *The Assault on Truth: Boris Johnson, Donald Trump and the emergence of a new moral barbarism*. London: Simon & Schuster, pp. 80–81.
15. https://committees.parliament.uk/oralevidence/2249/pdf/#page=29& zoom=page-fit,-541,843.
16. *The Observer*, 26 June 2021. Accessed 29 March 2021.
17. Ariely, D. (2008) *Predicably Irrational: The Hidden Forces That Shape Our Decisions*. New York: Harper Collins, p. 201. In Haidt (2012), p. 97.

2

Metaphors of the Pandemic: War

Introduction

The pandemic was framed in many different ways by journalists, politicians and other policy makers, sometimes as a 'forest fire', or as a 'rising tide'—but in this chapter I discuss the dominant 'war' frame—words such as 'frontline', 'Blitz' or 'invisible enemy'—and in the following chapter I discuss the 'fire' frame and the 'force of nature' frame. At the end of this chapter, I discuss some of the metaphors used in personal accounts by people who have suffered from Covid-19 and who mix various metaphors when describing their experience. I compare the Coronavirus pandemic with earlier accounts of the plague—such as those offered by Daniel Defoe in his *Journal of the Plague Year* and Albert Camus in *The Plague* that also show evidence of the 'war' frame. For each frame I discuss illustrations from the British press using the Nexis database and the findings of an online survey in which respondents undertook an empirical task designed to gauge how far their behaviour was influenced by different metaphors. Respondents were given three vignettes about coronavirus that varied only as regards to these 3 metaphor frames ('war, 'fire' and 'force of nature'), they were also given a vignette that described the same

© The Author(s), under exclusive license to Springer Nature Switzerland AG 2021
J. Charteris-Black, *Metaphors of Coronavirus*,
https://doi.org/10.1007/978-3-030-85106-4_2

events but without metaphors, i.e. literally. They were asked to rank five possible personal responses to the pandemic on a scale of importance ranging from the most to the least important. These responses varied in how far they were libertarian, or otherwise, for example at the extreme ends of the scale, people should either 'carry on life as normal' (most libertarian) or they should 'put their households into complete quarantine' (least libertarian). They were also invited to comment on the language used in the vignettes. But I will begin the chapter by discussing how, why and when journalists, politicians and even medical experts inevitably found themselves using 'war' related metaphors.

The War Frame

The sense of crisis that enveloped Britain with the onset of the pandemic made war the natural way of framing the experience. The exigencies of the situation demanded instant awareness that this was the greatest crisis since the Second World War and metaphor was crucial in creating acknowledgment of this reality and exhorting a concerted public response. There was an urgency to communicate the scale of the crisis because of the need for a massive political, social and economic response that would affect every aspect of life. As nations started to close down their economies, and sometimes their borders, and direct every possible resource towards care for patients suffering from Covid-19, it was perhaps inevitable that an analogy would be made in public discourse with a wartime situation. This is because 'war' serves as the most prototypical crisis requiring concerted social effort with life and death outcomes in situations where there are two sides with competing strategies. Unlike a flood, a volcano, a meteor strike, or other disasters caused by inanimate entities, a virus is a form of semi-animate entity that has a strategy: it can reproduce its DNA within its host. Although not fully alive, it is a parasite that competes with the life of the host DNA and adapts its strategies to the resistance it meets from human antibodies. The competitive nature of human and viral strategies combined with the destructive potential of Covid-19 therefore makes the framing of the efforts against the virus as a 'war' better motivated than it would be if we spoke about a 'war' against a volcano, a meteor strike or even climate change.

Coronavirus threatened to overwhelm the NHS in the United Kingdom because the government had been slow to introduce Lockdown measures and was reluctant to close down its borders thereby aggravating the crisis and making the scenario even more warlike as 'casualties' mounted. Having left everything too late, and seeking to escape blame, the British government described its policies using the language of war: a 'strategy' was developed with four 'tactical' aims: Contain—Delay—Research—Mitigate. The implementation of this strategy involved the construction of emergency 'field hospitals', deployment of an 'army' of health workers to 'fight' in 'the frontline'. They had to be 'equipped' as well as they could and provided with whatever 'weapons' were available. Had the government been better prepared, and the sense of crisis lesser, perhaps a frame other than war might have been possible. As it was, a wartime communications policy was initiated with daily press briefings attended by the Prime Minister, government ministers and advisers from 16th March 2020. Given such unpreparedness surely it would have been highly surprising if the crisis had *not* been framed as war?

> "We must act like any wartime government," declares Boris Johnson, sonorously channelling Churchill as he brings in measures "unprecedented since World War Two". The chancellor, Rishi Sunak, agrees: "We have never, in peacetime, faced an economic fight like this one." Britain is at war with "an invisible enemy," says the health secretary Matt Hancock. Dame Vera Lynn, still the forces' sweetheart at 103, exhorts a nation once again to embrace the spirit of the Blitz, "when we all pulled together".[1]

Many researchers acknowledge the inevitability of this: "the war frame is an effective way of grabbing people's attention and focusing it on the target problem; the fear evoked by war metaphors also makes them memorable and enduring... This fear can motivate people to pay attention, change their beliefs, and take action about important social issues."[2] However, some have criticized 'war' metaphors arguing that they were a reversion to a well-established and highly familiar discourse that was not effective because it emphasised tackling the *effects* of Covid19 without addressing the underlying *causes* of the pandemic.[3] Much of the antagonism towards war metaphors is because they are viewed as divisive as they assume a dichotomy between 'them' and 'us' which is an inappropriate perspective when unity is desired. However, in a study of the *China Daily*, (Yu, 2021) argues that Covid-19 was framed by the newspaper, reflecting the arguments of President Xi Jinping, as a 'common enemy of mankind' and that other nations were framed as China's 'allies' in a struggle for world health, under the leadership of the World Health Organization. In this rhetoric the war frame encourages co-operation and solidarity rather than division. In a collectivist approach the primary 'enemy' is market-driven individualism since this detracts from the co-operation necessary to 'defeat' the virus.[4] JF Kennedy in his celebrated inaugural address had referred to both 'war' and 'disease' (along with 'tyranny and poverty') as the 'common enemies of man', so there is nothing inherently divisive about war metaphors.[5] If we view war and disease as the most typical forms of non-natural disaster, then each can always be employed to frame the other. There was therefore nothing especially novel about viewing a virus as an 'enemy'; Defoe used this metaphor in his *Journal of the Plague Year*, written in 1722 this was—an account of the 1666 Great Plague of London:

> A plague is a formidable *enemy*, and is armed with terrors that every man is not sufficiently fortified to resist or prepare to stand the shock against…Why else do they exact a quarantine of those who came into their harbours and ports from suspected places? Forty day is, one would think, too long for nature to struggle with such an *enemy* as this, and not *conquer* it or yield to it.[6]

It is likely that there are significant cultural and historical influences at work in determining how people react to 'war' metaphors. Where the national identity has been based around fighting a heroic war of defence against foreign invaders, there is likely to be a more positive response than in nations where war is associated with shame, either because of defeat or because of guilt surrounding the policies that have caused war. By definition war causes destruction, death and harm and therefore disrupts the moral frame of Care/Harm even when enforced by considerations of Fairness ('Just War') or group Loyalty. I would therefore agree with Musolff (2021):

> …uses of the PANDEMIC-AS-WAR metaphor fulfil different rhetorical and argumentative functions: a) to rally support, b) to frame a narrative that explains developments in public health management and c) to justify specific policies. In view of such multi-functionality of metaphorical scenarios, some of the 'blanket criticism' of all occurrences of WAR and FIGHTING terminology appears to be unjustified.[7]

There is nothing inherently wrong or immoral about 'war' metaphors especially when they encourage unity and co-ordination against a common enemy of mankind, which seems to be the undeniable status accorded to Covid-19. Rather like addressing a stranger as 'brother' or 'sister', war metaphors can be linguistic strategies that create shared identities around shared purposes. Of course, they can also be used for self-aggrandizement by nationalist leaders seeking to eliminate democratic opponents, so we need to consider how, when, with what intention, and to what effect, war metaphors are employed when evaluating their ideological import. We need to consider the evolution of metaphor frames over a period of time according to shifting political goals. Silaški and Đurović confirm that "It has been well attested in the literature that some earlier health crises, such as AIDS, Ebola, SARS, bird flu, etc. were also perceived as warfare (Joffe & Haarhoff, 2002; Larson et al., 2005; Nerlich & Halliday, 2007; Sontag, 1989; Wallis & Nerlich, 2005)".[8]

Nor was the war framing an especially English metaphor; in English translations of Camus's *The Plague*, the narrator informs us of his doubts that forty days would be long enough to conquer an 'enemy' such as the plague:

> But, generally speaking, the epidemic was *in retreat* all along *the line*; the official communiques, which had at first encouraged no more than shadowy, half-hearted hopes, now confirmed the popular belief that the *victory was won* and *the enemy abandoning his positions*. Really, however, it is doubtful if this could be called a *victory*. All that could be said was that the

disease seemed to be leaving as unaccountably as it had come. Our *strategy* had not changed, but whereas yesterday it had obviously failed, today it seemed *triumphant*. Indeed, one's chief impression was that the epidemic had *called a retreat* after reaching all its objectives; it had, so to speak, achieved its purpose.[9]

It is part of the mythology of war that it will all be over soon, and yet it rarely is, and, as shown in the italicized metaphors, Camus captures the self-deception and illusory nature of 'victory' against the 'enemy', that is typified in Defoe's optimism.

Writing in *The Conversation*, David Hunter, A Professor of Epidemiology, provided a casebook illustration of how the war frame could be employed as an explanatory heuristic for critical reflection on the British response to the pandemic:

> The fight against COVID-19 has launched a thousand military metaphors in the British press. The "the greatest challenge since the Second World War" "the *frontline*", the virus is an "*invisible enemy*" and so forth. Us citizens feel besieged and under threat as we *retreat* to our foxholes.
>
> If this is a war, how is Britain doing? The *frontline troops* are running out of protective gear (PPE), *ammunition* (beds) and heavy *equipment* (ventilators). *Supply lines are stretched thin*. Meanwhile, the country's leadership—the prime minister, secretary of state for health and the chief medical officer—are self-isolated in their *bunkers* where they cannot be functioning at 100%....
>
> What do we need? We need the PPE and ventilators to reach the *troops* at the right time. But we also need reliable *intelligence* on the *enemy's movements*—we need to be able to test for the virus, and to test for past infection and current presumed immunity. We need these tests at the *front line* to work out who should be, and who should not be, in the *trenches*. We need the tests for the civilian *army*—to decide who can safely supply the elderly and infirm, staff the nursing and care homes, who can "*dig on for victory*" by maintaining the chain of food and essentials, and who should continue to isolate at home.[10]

The writer explores the material aspects of war but also the psychological importance of leadership and of morale. The war frame enables him to highlight a comprehensive strategy for what needed to be done and argues for the complete mobilisation of material and social resources necessary for a response to a pandemic.

But it is not only the social response to crisis that invites the 'war' frame, it is also employed to describe the process of infection, as, when appearing on Channel 5s Jeremy Vine show, Dr Sarah Jarvis argued in the context of comparing cancer treatment with Covid-19 that although she had "always been in favour of people having choice …A big difference here is that *breathing is an offensive weapon* if you are infected with Covid".[11] The comment received much criticism online for its hyperbole but war metaphors are commonly employed to describe the reaction of the body itself when struggling with disease and infection. Consider the italicized metaphors in this extract that occurs early on in a book that gives a historical overview of ten major pandemics during the twentieth century:

> When a parasitic organism meets a susceptible host for the first time, it *triggers* an *arms race* between the pathogen and the host's immune system. Having never encountered the pathogen before, the immune system is initially *blindsided* and takes time to *mobilize* its *defences* and *launch* a *counterattack*. With nothing to stop it, the pathogen *tears* through the host's tissue, *invading* cells and multiplying at will… From a Darwinian point of view, however, the parasite does not want to *kill* its host; its primary objective is to survive long enough to *escape* and infect a new susceptible. In other words, the death of the host is a bad *strategy* for a parasite…A far better survival *strategy* over the long term is to evolve in the other direction, toward avirulence, resulting in an infection that is mild or barely detectable in the host.[12]

We find that the dynamic relationship of a parasite with its host over time is captured by at least a dozen 'war' metaphors based around the central idea of 'strategy' which derives from the Greek *strategia*, 'generalship'. It is not just the conflict between two entities that relies on the 'war' metaphor but the whole scenario of planning, tactics and success: it is because the virus has a strategy that the body needs to develop one of its own if it is to survive. It is almost natural to speak of 'fighting' an infection, and we encourage our immune system to 'attack' or 'kill' alien viruses that might 'destroy' our health. We do not at first consider these viruses to be our 'allies', but eventually we 'protect' ourselves against them by introducing a 'double agent' in the form of a vaccine. A typical vaccine is a small amount of that which we wish to protect ourselves against, the metaphorical 'enemy', but it is administered in such a finely tuned quantity that it works rather like a spy: it deceives our body into an attacking mode by pretending it is one of the 'enemy'. Immunology is all about triggering the body's *own protective responses* in favour of the host and against the intruding virus. We might watch animations depicting our 'blue armies' deflecting the alien 'red army' from latching onto our native 'blue' cells. There may be other more technical and sophisticated ways of describing how immunity develops but, at least for now, it seems that 'fighting an invasion' is probably the most cognitively accessible.

Rejection of the War Metaphor

In a recent account the author argues that the government systematically weaponised fear against the British population through drawing on behavioural psychology and that war framing was part of a more general propaganda operation to instil fear, and thereby control, the British population.[13] However, it would have been surprising if the government had not drawn on all disciplines, including behavioural psychology to persuade the population of the urgency of the situation. More literal language would perhaps have been more honest, but given that their messages were in competition with the hyperbole and metaphor of the British media, would they have been listened to if metaphor was avoided? Perhaps a more insightful question might be whether the war frame was a good one? While there were ways in which the situation in March 2020 was similar to war, there are some others respects in which the Coronavirus pandemic was *not* at all like a war, at least one such as the older generation in Britain had experienced and had been embedded in the social rituals of Remembrance Days, war memorials and myths about Blitz heroism. In a war there are identifiable human combatants in 'Them' and 'Us' roles; yet here the enemy were tiny bundles of genes wrapped up in coats of protein so small they require an electron microscope to be visible, so if this were a war *where* exactly was this enemy? Typically, war involves an overseas enemy—another nation state—which state was it? For Donald Trump it was clearly China, and for China it must therefore be the US. But most nations exchanged knowledge and resources in an effort to create a global alliance represented by the WHO. This was more a war against an alien invader than one between nations, hence an outbreak of cultural interest in zombie moves.

War usually entails overseas combat and the transportation of resources to a distant frontline and interruption of supplies; yet here it was quite different, people stayed at home and many were sent food and supplies financed by the government's furlough scheme.[14] This 'war' was being fought entirely on the 'Home Front'—more like a guerrilla war then, but not a Civil War. And what of the victims? Usually, war casualties are fit young men whereas in this 'war' they were the oldest, most obese, physically most vulnerable and most likely to come from black and minority ethnic backgrounds. War involves a massive sensory overload: a great deal of noise, bombs and explosions, the shrieks of the wounded, bright flashes of light and, for those physically present, the stench of burning tyres or burning flesh. Yet this 'war' was characterised by its silence as people were told to 'Stay Home' and traffic practically ceased, the only sounds were the endless ambulance sirens shuffling the infected to hospital. The lights we could now see were the stars that reappeared over cities that had previously been obscured by pollution and the smell was the returning scent of greenery as nature restored itself: this was some strange war that instead of ruining nature was improving it! During actual wartime the British avoid expression of intense feeling but during the pandemic there was endless discussion of wellbeing. During wartime people cluster together for solidarity, safety or reassurance, in pubs, homes or bunkers, but now they were instructed to avoid others, to stay as isolated as possible and avoid contact even with the Amazon delivery worker. Those who chatted together on street corners had become a fifth column of potential traitors. In war people celebrate victory but nobody knew what victory would look like in the case of a pandemic. In many crucial respects, socially and psychologically, this disaster was quite unlike a war!

There were other reasons why the 'war' metaphor was rejected. One of these was that the metaphor itself was a cliché and like a tired elastic band had lost its tension through overuse, as a journalist noted:

> In any case, the 'war' analogy has been rendered meaningless after overuse by governments and campaigners, long before the coronavirus struck.
>
> The war on drugs, the war on obesity, the war on poverty, the war on plastic, the war on saturated fats ... the list is almost endless.
>
> In the case of the coronavirus, the politicians are not just using it as a metaphor but as an exact comparison with the British people's struggle in 1939–1945. It really isn't at all like that...The current crisis is nothing like that (the Blitz). Our homes are not threatened with destruction. The very existence of our country is not at stake, as it was then. This is not a war, or anything like it.[15]

Some authors combined a criticism of the war frame with the proposal for an alternative one:

> It's time leaders levelled with us that this is more like the Aids crisis than a military conflict. There is nothing worse than a bad metaphor in a crisis. Just as Blair and Bush declared a "war on terror" in the wake of 9/11, Trump is "mobilising" against a mysterious "Chinese virus". Meanwhile Britain has created a "War Cabinet" and instructed its Home Front to stay indoors while invoking the Blitz spirit....Perhaps they (the government) might have done this by framing the outbreak of Covid-19 as more similar to the Aids crisis than the Second World War. That is, to explain that a nasty new virus is suddenly in our midst and that scientists have limited knowledge of how it spreads, how to cure it or whether it might mutate.[16]

Of course, since AIDS was a viral infection, it is questionable whether using it to understand Coronavirus would really be a metaphor, or if it would have been any less frightening. The writer goes to note that "war-time bluster" is unrealistically raising expectations:

> The media's desperate search for the Government's secret weapon to blast the virus—before finally settling on the idea that the silver bullet must be mass testing, and skewering ministers and PHE over their related failings—being a striking example.

The author here seems more concerned with avoiding the hyperbole of war and to be taking a counter-position against the well-established war frame. Other commentators, such as Robert Fisk, who had witnessed and reported on many wars, preferred a more balanced account that acknowledged that there were arguments in favour of, and opposed to, war metaphors:

> I do have some sympathy with the metaphors of war. Doctors, nurses, ambulance drivers and paramedics are indeed on a "frontline". For not only are they literally fighting to save the lives of others; they are also, in a sense, coming under fire as they mind their posts—because the virus is shooting back at them, infecting them and in some cases killing them. They are in danger of being eliminated by an enemy which they are trying to destroy. Although we should not, perhaps, forget that we, too, are on a front line—it is the "wounded" among us that the doctors are trying to save....I'm less easy, though, about the constant references to the Blitz spirit—not just because the Blitz was an invention of a certain nation which is now fighting the same "war" against coronavirus as us, but because these allusions lend themselves to dangerous exaggeration.

What Fisk illustrates here is awareness of the agency of the virus: it 'is shooting back' which implies that it has a strategy. So, he does not reject the war frame in general, but at the end of the extract he rejects metaphors from particular wars—London's experience of the Second World War—because they are too historically restricted and no longer resonate with younger audiences. I found some support for this point of view in some research I undertook that elicited comments about the war frame and is described in more detail in the next section. A few respondents described their reaction to the Blitz used as a metaphor:

> While the Blitz spirit/war image one (which is somewhat similar to the language actually used by Boris Johnson) made me roll my eyes a bit.

> The Blitz language is just annoying. Happy to have a conversation about the second world war and its time period any day of the week, but not so happy to understand everything that happens today through its meaning making frameworks.

The use of the Blitz is likely to cause greater concern among older generations, perhaps? This could mean they are more likely to see the severity of
the issue.

For these respondents the Blitz was simply not relatable and Blitz metaphors no longer seemed relevant to what they were experiencing. During
the Blitz citizens were exhorted to blackout their windows to prevent
them from being used to target bombing raids. By contrast, in the pandemic many put coloured lights, attractive silhouetted craft works, and
beautifully painted 'NHS' rainbows in their windows. It may be because
of a growing awareness that media commentators gradually withdrew
from using war metaphors as the pandemic progressed. War metaphors
were used early on to create a sense of urgency and therefore to enforce
compliance with constraints on personal liberties. But as the pandemic
progressed, they not only became more cliched, they also no longer
seemed to evoke empathetic responses and their confrontational tone
seemed likely to disrupt social cohesion: if this was a war, then the
only two sides were life and death.

Empirical Research & Analysis

I undertook a search of the theme of 'Coronaviruses' in the 'UK National
Newspapers' section of the Nexis database for the period 1st February
2020 to 28th February 2021. The following table shows the frequency of
a sample of the war lexicon over this one-year period (omitting July–
September for reasons of space). The numbers indicate the number of
separate stories in which there is at least one use of a word from the lexical
field of 'war' rather than the total number of uses (so where there is repetition of a word in the same story the total numbers of uses would
increase). I have not searched every word in context to see if it was metaphoric, but since the stories were all on the theme of Coronavirus rather
than 'war' it is likely that they were. A similar procedure is taken with the
other tables throughout the book.

Table 2.1 only shows a sample of the lexical field of 'war' which could
also have included words such as: arms, to attack, to beat, to combat, to

Table 2.1 The lexical field of 'war' in the British Press (2020–2021)

	2020								2021	
	Feb	Mar	April	May	June	Oct	Nov	Dec	Jan	Feb
Battle	481	5278	6810	4392	3237	3059	2719	2340	3098	2369
War	580	5191	5738	4412	2865	2569	2255	1925	2450	2246
Frontline	174	3881	7181	3536	1627	920	1105	1623	2450	1491
Troops	77	798	573	447	682	323	436	350	518	284
Bomb	75	502	587	500	334	368	309	304	331	247
Blitz	38	440	347	289	220	165	173	129	271	225
Surrender	19	130	160	291	120	159	117	88	102	113
Invisible enemy/ killer	5	234	316	135	67	28	29	25	14	24
Siege	8	95	106	82	65	56	49	44	185	70
Total	1457	16,549	21,818	14,084	9217	7647	7192	6828	9419	7069

defeat, to deploy, to defend, Hitler, to invade, lines of defence, to repel, to wage, weapon etc. but the sample here allows comparison of changes in the frequency of war lexis longitudinally over a period of time.

Table 2.1 shows that the lexical field of war increased exponentially with the onset of the pandemic; between February and March 'war' words increased by more than tenfold. They continued to rise by a third again in April, then, though still high, from May onwards they declined (with the exception of 'troops'); the use of 'frontline' fell by three quarters between April and June and 'battle' decreased by more than half as the sense of crisis dissipated. Although all the 'war' words rose again with the second wave in January 2021, they declined in February as the sense of crisis reduced. The questionable 'Blitz' metaphor was half what it had been the previous March as it had now become a rather conventional metaphor used mainly by the popular media. The 'Blitz' metaphor featured in 787 different stories in March and April 2020, but often with a degree of mitigation and explanation as to why it was being used:

> The term "Blitz spirit" is tired and overused, yet it does sum up the attitude required in times such as these—when people, even more than usual, need to go about their business with an eye to the common good.[17]

Even *The Daily Telegraph* was taking a somewhat qualified view of the Blitz spirit metaphor:

> Evoking the Blitz spirit during the coronavirus pandemic is more complex than it first appears. That spirit is one of the cornerstones of our national myth, but like all myths it contains as much falsehood as truth. Crime rates went up more than 50 per cent during the war, with looting rife and a thriving black market. During the eight months of the Blitz, people were often panicked, and sometimes had to be forced into shelters. Show me a population prepared to obey a government without question and I will show you a country not worth living in.
>
> Above all, the five words most closely associated with the Blitz spirit— "keep calm and carry on"—were rarely used at the time. ... But it is in these very shifts that we can harness the deeper meaning of the "Blitz spirit". We must stay resilient, not give up hope and remember that this too will pass.[18]

There is then some indication that the views of the questionnaire respondents matched with those of Robert Fisk and other journalists. It was a metaphor that had an increasingly limited appeal to a declining elderly population.

The same progression from novelty to fatigue occurred with the 'invisible enemy', at the onset of the pandemic following the leadership of Matt Hancock it had become the standard metaphor used by those in the 'frontline':

> Joan Glen, 61, is doing gruelling 12-hour shifts wearing full PPE equipment as a theatre nurse treating Covid-19 patients. The mother-of-three who lives near Chester says the circumstances are eerily similar to her experience treating badly injured soldiers in wartorn Afghanistan. It is *just like a war* here in our hospitals, just another *kind of war*,' she said in an exclusive interview with MailOnline. It was frightening out there and it's frightening here now—this is *like a war* but this is *an invisible enemy.* Out in Afghanistan we were fighting the Taliban but this is a virus—you can't see it but it's deadly.'[19]

In fact the speaker was echoing the Health Secretary who had announced in a speech on 1st April 2020: "If the past few weeks have shown us anything, it's that we are steadfast as a country in our resolve to defeat this invisible killer."[20] The expression 'invisible killer' occurred in 383 news stories in the year from 1st March 2020, as compared with only 52 stories the preceding year. Evidently, the expression was intended to arouse the emotion of fear: this was not just a killer, but one that would creep up on you without you knowing. The invisible nature of this animate danger was also something that Defoe had commented in relation to the Plague, when describing what later became known as 'miasma theory':

> …likewise the opinion of others, who talk of infection being carried on by the air only, by carrying with it vast numbers of insects and *invisible creatures*, who enter into the body with the breath, or even at the pores with the air, and there generate or emit most acute poisons, or poisonous ovae or eggs, which mingle themselves with the blood, and so infect the body.

The word 'creatures' here is quite general but it is their tiny size that enables them to enter at the pores that is salient. But journalists were tiring of the 'invisible enemy' by February 2021 its use was much lower than it had been in the first wave and more restricted to the popular press.

> THE tributes to Captain Sir Tom Moore, following his death with Covid at the age of 100, have been heartfelt and deeply moving. The remarkable old soldier fought fascism in the Second World War then became a beacon in our current *battle against an invisible enemy*.[21]

It is worth noting that whereas some of the war lexicon increased in the early months of 2021, words such as 'battle', 'war', 'frontline' and 'Blitz' were more frequent in the press in January 2021 than they had been in November 2020, this was not the case with 'invisible enemy/killer'. This suggests that as the virus became better known war metaphors became more conventional and attempts to activate emotions such as fear, that politicians believed to be necessary, were now through metaphors of physical combat such as boxing or wrestling. I discuss these in terms of physical force in the next chapter. The effect is to reduce the sense of impending disaster and to heighten the sense of embodied struggle against an opponent.

But what is the effect of such metaphors on people's reasoning? In a much-cited research study informants were given a situation in which an imaginary city was experiencing an outbreak of crime. They then investigated how different metaphor frames influenced people's reasoning about solving the problem of crime in an imaginary city and found that the type of solution they proposed depended on how crime was framed:[22]

> We asked people to imagine a "virus infecting a city" or a "wild beast preying on a city" and then to describe the best way to solve the problem that they had imagined. Participants who imagined a "virus infecting the city" universally suggested investigating the source of the virus and implementing social reforms and prevention measures to decrease the spread of the virus. That is, they wanted to know where the virus was coming from, whether the city could develop a vaccine and how the virus was spreading. They also wanted to institute educational campaigns to inform residents about how to avoid or deal with the virus and encourage residents to follow better hygiene practices. Participants who imagined a "wild beast preying on a city" universally suggested capturing the beast and then killing or caging it. They wanted to organize a hunting party or hire animal control specialists to track down the beast and stop it from ravaging the city.

When crime was framed as a virus, they proposed socially liberal solutions that addressed the causes of crime, but when it was framed as a beast, they proposed socially illiberal solutions such as killing or caging the beast. The contrast in attitudinal responses was attributed to the choice of metaphor frame. This research found that metaphor needed to be introduced early in the vignettes to have such a framing effect. In the empirical part of my research, instead of creating an imaginary scenario I used a real one—the pandemic—to gauge the effect of metaphor on attitudes towards different behaviours during the pandemic. Respondents to an online survey were asked to read an invented narrative or 'vignette' (like the one above) that included approximately 8 'war' related metaphors,[23] these could be words or phrases and are shown in italics below (the version used by respondents did not italicize the metaphors):

War Vignette

Imagine it is 16 March 2020, 3 months after Coronavirus *broke out* in China. Italy is badly *hit* as the *biological war* against the virus as it *marches* across Europe. In the UK, Prime Minister Boris Johnson *devises his plan of attack* by *deploying* retired healthcare workers for *the frontline.* 251 new cases have been reported today and as the nation's death toll reaches 35. While Cheltenham races were given the go ahead, Johnson now calls for *Blitz Spirit,* instructing non-key workers to work from home and advising the public to avoid pubs and restaurants.

They were also asked to read the following vignette that is the same length and in which the same propositional content is expressed literally (i.e. avoiding metaphor):

Literal Vignette

Imagine it is 16 March 2020, 3 months after the Coronavirus pandemic began in China. Italy reports an increase in cases as the situation worsens across Europe. In the UK, Prime Minister Boris Johnson plans emergency procedures, calling on retired healthcare workers to prepare to return to work. 251 new cases have been reported today and as the nation's death toll reaches 35. While Cheltenham races were given the go ahead, Johnson now calls for compliance, instructing non-key workers to work from home and advising the public to avoid pubs and restaurants.

I then asked respondents to rank five statements relating to their personal decisions in order of their importance on a scale of high importance to low importance. The personal decisions were based on various aspects of government guidance and were as follows:

1. Carry on life as normal.
2. Go out as normal but begin 2m social distancing everywhere.

3. Limit outings to 1 hour a day for essential trips and exercise only.
4. Strictly limit outings to essential trips only.
5. Put their household into complete quarantine.

These statements were intended to reflect how much individuals were prepared to modify their behaviours to protect themselves and society from the spread of the virus. For example, option 1 does not involve any change of behaviour and is the most libertarian, whereas option 5 requires the highest level of behavioural change and is the least libertarian. The vignettes were then modified with different metaphor frames, 'fire', 'force of nature' etc. and I will report on these in the following chapter. Respondents were invited to comment in general terms on the vignettes after having completed the rank ordering exercise with the question: "Do you have any other thoughts or comments on any of the language used in any of these accounts?"

A total of 75 respondents completed the war vignette and 71 completed the literal vignettes and 38 commented on some aspect of language in the vignettes. The findings for the two vignettes are shown in Tables 2.2 and 2.3:

Statistical analysis involved comparing the ranking of each of the 5 responses separately for the two vignettes; for example, the rankings for response 1 'Carry on life as normal' after reading the war vignette were compared with the rankings for this option after reading the literal vignette. For most of the responses there was no significant difference

Table 2.2 Responses to the war vignette

Behaviours	1st rank	2nd rank	3rd rank	4th rank	5th rank
Carry on life as normal	3	0	1	5	66
Go out as normal but begin 2M social distancing everywhere	2	8	30	35	0
Limit outings to 1 hour a day, for essential trips and exercise only	14	34	23	4	0
Strictly limit outings to essential trips only	35	23	11	6	0
Put their household into complete quarantine	21	10	10	25	9

Table 2.3 Responses to the literal vignette

Behaviours	1st rank	2nd rank	3rd rank	4th rank	5th rank
Carry on life as normal	4	1	1	5	60
Go out as normal but begin 2M social distancing everywhere	5	6	35	25	0
Limit outings to 1 hour a day, for essential trips and exercise only	18	40	9	4	0
Strictly limit outings to essential trips only	35	20	9	6	1
Put their household into complete quarantine	9	4	17	31	10

between the two vignettes suggesting that respondents' judgements of the relative importance of different behavioural responses during the pandemic had already been formed prior to reading the vignettes and so were not significantly influenced by them. In contrast to the earlier study that was based on an imaginary city and did not relate to a current real world crisis, my vignettes related to informants' everyday lived experience of an actual situation. People had already formed views about how to respond to the pandemic that were unlikely to be shifted by metaphor. The comments of several respondents support this interpretation:

> Personally, I feel the wording of the accounts doesn't impact my policy decisions massively. My exposure to what I was seeing as a healthcare clinician at the time shaped my views more. In terms of media reports, I have been more focused on the content and the facts, although I'm aware that language has the potential to impose a bias depending on the source.

> I did not feel that the language used changed my view on what policies I saw as most important. I feel like that might be because I have already been desensitised to scary language about the virus. Perhaps looking at the fear response provoked by different newspaper headlines which use different metaphors could have had more of an obvious affect on me.

> Well clearly the language has been changed in each of the versions. I can see that the language in some is purposively inflammatory etc. I was aware of the differences in all the versions but in no way swayed by this. I have pro-

cessed the information on Covid19, I have read the various scientific accounts and have made my own mind up on the best course of action.

Emotive language but had no effect because we know what happened already and would have strongly held personal beliefs about delayed government action.

Only that I don't think the language used had any effect on my ranking decisions—which were all made based on what I already know about the situation with coronavirus/COVID, and different governments' response to it.

However, there was one response for which a statistically significant difference was identified—this was the option that required the *highest level* of behaviour change: "Put their household into complete quarantine". This was ranked as most important by more of those after reading the 'war' vignette than it was after their reading the literal vignette and the difference was statistically significant. A Chi-Square test showed there was a significant relationship between the war vignette and the 'complete quarantine' response, $x2 (1, N = 75) = 9.78, p = 0.044311$ which makes the result significant ($p > 0.05$). There was only one comment that acknowledged the view that war metaphors were persuasive:

When the language was quite emotive by references to wartime, it makes you feel like it's community effort. Everyone is in it together.

A possible interpretation of the discrepancy between the comments on the impact of metaphors and the ranking of responses to the pandemic is that the effect of metaphor is largely unconscious. In the original study the researchers found that:

When given the opportunity to identify the most influential aspect of the crime report, participants (in all four studies that include a metaphoric frame) ignore the metaphor. Instead, they cite the crime statistics (which are the same in both conditions) as being influential in their reasoning.

In a similar way it may be that the informants in this study prefer not to admit to the influence of the war frame because it is not one that they believe to be positively perceived. In addition to the negative comments concerning the Blitz, a couple of comments indicate this negative perception of the war frame:

> For me the message is the same regardless of some of the language being obviously inflammatory or fear mongering referencing war metaphors.
> …using too military language is not appropriate to a virus.

However, as with the earlier study, what respondents consciously claim may not accord with the unconscious influence of metaphor frames on their behaviour. This survey, larger than the original one, therefore shows that framing the pandemic as war may have actively heightened the awareness of the danger presented by coronavirus and that this awareness heightened the emotion of fear and may have had an unconscious influence on their beliefs: metaphor may have made it more likely that people would support a policy of complete quarantine.

Mixed Metaphors

Mixed metaphors occur when a metaphor from one frame such as 'war' occurs alongside a metaphor from a quite different frame such as 'nature', 'journey' or 'fire'. Mixed metaphors have generally been criticised as indicative of poor style, or even worse, poor thought—instances of cognitive error—however this view has recently been challenged by specialists in the field.[24] In this section I show some empirical evidence of their impact on audiences and their emotional power in conveying the experience of suffering from Covid-19.

Given the potential impact of mixed metaphors I also included in the empirical research described above a vignette reporting on the pandemic that used mixed metaphors to gauge their effect on the informants for the online survey described above. This is the vignette that was used:

Mixed Metaphor Vignette

Imagine it is 16 March 2020, 3 months after the *unwelcome* Coronavirus *barged* into China. Italy is in *overdrive* as the virus *hacks its way* into Europe. In the UK, Prime Minister Boris Johnson *pulls the trigger, ejecting* retired healthcare workers out into the *hurricane.* 251 new cases have been reported today and as the nation's death toll reaches 35. While Cheltenham races were given the go ahead, Johnson now calls for *team spirit,* instructing non-key workers to work from home and advising the public to avoid pubs and restaurants.

Here, rather than coming from a single frame, the metaphors are from the different semantic fields of 'hospitality', 'physical force', 'computing', 'war', 'weather', 'sports' etc. A total of 110 respondents completed the mixed metaphor vignette; this is higher than for the 'war' or the literal vignette as it occurred earlier in the survey before a fatigue factor had set in. One of the difficulties with the research design was that due to time constraints I was only able to conduct a single survey covering several different metaphor frames (some of which are not shown here) whereas ideally a series of separate surveys would have been conducted over a longer period. The responses to the five statements ranking the order of their importance of various responses are shown in Table 2.4:

There was some indication that informants shifted to less libertarian responses in response to mixed metaphors as 55% ranked the strictest, least libertarian responses (essential trips only and complete quarantine)

Table 2.4 Responses to the mixed metaphor vignette

Behaviours	1st rank	2nd rank	3rd rank	4th rank	5th rank
Carry on life as normal	2	2	1	4	101
Go out as normal but begin 2M social distancing everywhere	10	6	41	52	1
Limit outings to 1 hour a day, for essential trips and exercise only	29	50	27	4	0
Strictly limit outings to essential trips only	51	41	15	2	1
Put their household into complete quarantine	18	11	26	48	7

as one of their two most important priorities, whereas the figure was only 48% after reading the literal vignette (it was 59% for the war vignette). However, these results were not statistically significant, reinforcing the point that in a contemporary real life crisis any conscious political viewpoints are formed by a wide range of social and attitudinal responses that are not directly, or consciously, influenced by metaphor. However, that does not exclude the possibility of their having a powerful unconscious effect and some of the responses suggest that the respondents were partially aware of the power of mixed metaphors:

> Different overall messages—pull the community together like in the war, fear of a horrible plague etc.

> Some of the accounts portray a calmer message than the others and felt more 'factual'. Some accounts felt fearful and used more dramatic language. These more fearful accounts made me feel like I wanted the government and the public to take stronger action!

We are not always full conscious of what makes us most afraid, fear by its nature is often of something on the hinterland of our consciousness, and it may be that metaphor frames such as 'war' and mixed metaphors work indirectly, especially through the language of public communication.

When people are faced by personal crisis, they are often compelled to use mixed metaphors when reflecting on the emotional chaos of this experience and this seems to have been the case in some of the personal accounts of sufferers of Covid-19. When embodied experience is beyond our control, this experience is often expressed in language that initially appears incoherent or dislocated because the metaphors are mixed. However, on reflection, this mixing of metaphor may be expressing at the emotional level the chaotic nature of the lived experience of Covid-19. In earlier research I have found that feelings of loss of control were a central theme in accounts by both people experiencing depression and in those who have experienced chronic pain. In both these other illness conditions speakers mixed their metaphors to emphasise the intensity of the embodied experience by representing the condition as one where they were *out of control*.[25] The greater the semantic divergence of metaphor source domains (for example 'clothes' and 'fire'), the more intense the embodied experience of mental suffering and the less the agency of the person experiencing the condition. The loss of control that is expressed in first-person accounts with apparently incoherent metaphors may be shown to be highly coherent when analysed symbolically since they communicate what Frank (1995) describes as 'Chaos narratives'. An analysis of accounts of Covid-19 sufferers that I found on various web sources showed similar findings to the ones I uncovered in more controlled interview conditions for sufferers of depression and of chronic pain. The Covid accounts might start a description with a war frame and then morph into other metaphor frames to convey the emotionally disturbed nature of the experience. Consider how this happens in the following account of Stewart Boyle, a 64-year-old man who experienced Covid-19:

> It's quite subtle at first," he explains. "But then I would try to climb the stairs and be wheezing *like an old man*. Soon I didn't have the ability to exercise or move at all. The virus *was attacking* my lungs and I was *losing the capacity to fight back*." "It was *like something out of a movie*," he says. "I was wheeled into the '*red zone*' and there were loads of tests being carried out and swabs being taken. They thought I had coronavirus so they *upped* my oxygen. There were a couple of hours where I was *within a whisper of a very dark place* and I thought, 'maybe my time is up'. But I wanted to live.
>
> I could feel *the battle in my lungs* and *it required all my reserves to get through it.* The extra oxygen *gave my lungs a break* and gave me the added energy *to push out* the disease. The NHS staff were incredible, but all they can do is help you *fight the virus*. There's no vaccination or *magical potion* that can save you. It's about your own resilience.[26]

There is a high density of metaphors, but they are superficially incoherent because they are mixed. He starts with the war frame ('attacking' etc), then brings in a 'movie' frame then 2 other frames 'whisper' ('speech' frame) and 'dark place' (frame of 'light' and 'dark') before returning to the war frame with 'battle' and 'fight'; there is even the introduction of a 'magic' frame towards the end. But the point is that he is grabbing at different images to reflect an entirely consistent and coherent narrative: one of loss of control, which then leads him to 'fight back' against the illness. In this sense it is not a chaotic narrative at all but one that narrates a retrospective story about the experience of chaos brought on by a health condition.

Metaphor mixing in a narrative of chaotic experience does not necessarily draw on the war frame alone, as in the following, account by Connor Read, a 24-year-old man, that includes a range of metaphors to express the embodied experience of the long terms effects of the illness. There are 'fire' metaphors ('burning'); 'motion' metaphors ('come back', 'take …away'); and other creative metaphors to express the experience of either body parts (the lungs) or the whole body ('run over by a steamroller'):

> "This is no longer just a cold. I ache all over, my head is thumping, my eyes are *burning*, my throat is constricted," he wrote.
>
> He said his 'bones were aching' and he had a '*hacking* cough'.
>
> By day 11 he thought the flu had lifted, but admitted that it had *come* '*back* with a vengeance' the next day.
>
> "I'm sweating, *burning up*, dizzy and shivering. The television is on but I can't make sense of it. This is a *nightmare*," he said.
>
> I can't take more than *sips of air* and, when I breathe out, my lungs *sound like a paper bag being crumpled up*. This isn't right. I need to see a doctor.
>
> After a visit to the doctor and several hours of tests he said he was diagnosed with pneumonia.
>
> A few days later, the pneumonia had gone but he said he ached "as if *I've been run over by a steamroller*".
>
> My sinuses are agony, and my eardrums feel *ready to pop*. I know I shouldn't but I'm massaging my inner ear with cotton buds, trying to *take the pain away*.[27]

By switching between different metaphor frames, he expresses feelings of his lack of control over the experience and the intensity of symptoms that include bodily heat, breathing sounds, and pressure. The more forceful the semantic collision of semantically divergent metaphors ('a paper bag', 'a steamroller' etc.), the more intense the embodied experience of suffering, and the greater the agency of the cause of suffering (Covid-19) rather than that of the speaker. The clashing of source domains that occurs in mixed metaphor symbolically re-enacts the chaotic and disruptive experience that characterises the embodied experience of intense physical and psychological suffering. Consider the testimony of a 49-year-old woman, Elizabeth, in her account of Covid-19:

> At one point, I felt the most almighty pain in my chest, like I was being *compressed with slabs of concrete*. They told me it was the pneumonia *attacking* my lungs and they gave me a shot of morphine. That was followed by terrible *stabbing* pains in my stomach, as bad as *labour contractions*, and I cried out: "I can't take this anymore! I can't carry on!" By the time the pains subsided, I was almost delirious.[28]

Note how she shifts from the powerful image of 'slabs of concrete' to a war metaphor 'attack' before shifting on to other frames such as 'childbirth'. A similar use of semantically divergent images occurs in this account of the experience of Covid-19 by Robin Bowler, a 58-year-old man:

> Other times I was *floating in a circular motion inside a large natural bowl of thick green vegetation*, but try as I might, I could never *see the rim of the bowl* and the sky above.
>
> And all this time, the constant refrain of WHOOSH, HISS, WHOOSH, HISS, WHOOSH, HISS, dominating the weird version of consciousness that I found myself in. And a clear voice in my head then reminded me that I was *fighting for my life*.
>
> It said that I was in the *Staying Alive Factory*, and that if I wanted to survive, I needed to stay on this *noisy, uncomfortable, frightening production line*; and that alternatively, if I *fell off the production line*, I would not make it through. So that was it.[29]

His vivid narrative includes the powerful sensory image of a bowl of green vegetation, but then diverges to the very different image of the 'Staying Alive Factory', sandwiched between these two images is the 'fighting' metaphor. There is no superficial coherence to these metaphors, but it is precisely the chaotic 'circular motion' of his language that seems to convey feelings of loss of agency and dependency on others.

The expression of loss of agency through the mixing of images also occurs in articles that report on people's dreaming experience during the pandemic:

Meanwhile, others dream of losing control. In one such dream, the dreamer was held down by infected people who coughed on her. In another, the dreamer came across bands of people shooting at random strangers.[30]

The images of people being randomly shot at, or being coughed over by the infected, share the sense of experiencing an extreme loss of agency. It is also worth noting the diversity of the disaster images in accounts of dreams:

> There are earthquakes, tidal waves and tornadoes; every kind of uncontrollable disaster. But the biggest dream cluster is bugs; flying bugs attacking the dreamer, cockroaches swarming, masses of squirming worms.[31]

Here there is a switch from extreme weather conditions to bugs and creepie crawlies: what they share is that they echo biblical images of divine punishment and disaster. What Covid-19 patients have in common with everyone is that at times during the pandemic they needed to communicate the emotional experience of losing control, whether because of illness itself or through the imagined experience of catching Covid-19 when dreaming. What both types of account (illness narratives and dreams) share is that they draw on mixed metaphors to express the experience of a consciousness that is no longer in full control of the body. What I have suggested, and is hinted at by some of the survey respondents, is that the effect of metaphor is not always one of which we are fully conscious, and the evidence from accounts of dreams, as well those of sufferers of Covid-19, suggests that these unconscious experiences may be ones that are best expressed by mixed metaphors. Sometimes these metaphors include war imagery but at others, as here, they include fire and forces of nature -i.e. other disaster-related imagery; it is these metaphors that form the topic of the next chapter.

Notes

1. *thetimes.co.uk*, 20 March, 2020.
2. Flusberg, S. J., Matlock, T., & Thibodeau, P. H. (2018). War metaphors in public discourse. *Metaphor and Symbol*, *33*(1), 1–18. p. 7.

3. Oswick, C, Grant, D. & Oswick, R. (2020) Categories, Crossroads, Control, Connectedness, Continuity, and Change: A Metaphorical Exploration of COVID-19. *Journal of Applied Behavioural Science*, 56 (3), pp. 284–288.

4. Yu, Y. (2021) Legitimising a global fight for a shared future: A critical metaphor analysis of the reportage of COVID-19 in *China Daily*. In A. Musolff, R. Breeze, S. Vilar-Lluch and K. Kondo (eds.) *Pandemic and Crisis Discourse: Communicating COVID-19 and Public Health Strategy*. London: Bloomsbury. Chapter 14.

5. JF Kennedy referred to a "struggle against the common enemies of man: tyranny, poverty, disease and war itself".

6. http://www.gutenberg.org/files/376/376-h/376-h.htm. Accessed 29 March 2021.

7. Musolff, A. (2021) "War against COVID-19": Is the pandemic as war metaphor helpful or hurtful? In A. Musolff, R. Breeze, S. Vilar-Lluch and K. Kondo (eds.) *Pandemic and Crisis Discourse: Communicating COVID-19 and Public Health Strategy*. London: Bloomsbury. Chapter 18.

8. Joffe, H., & Haarhoff, G. (2002). Representations of far-flung illnesses: The case of Ebola in Britain. *Social Science & Medicine*, 54(6), 955–969.

   Larson, B. M., Nerlich, B., & Wallis, P. (2005). Metaphors and biorisks: The war on infectious diseases and invasive species. *Science Communication*, 26(3), 243–268.

   Nerlich, H., & Halliday, C. (2007). Avian flu: the creation of expectations in the interplay between science and the media. *Sociology of Health and Illness*, 29 (1): 46–65.

   Sontag, S. (1989). *Illness as metaphor and AIDS and its metaphors*. London/New York: Penguin Modern Classics.

   Wallis, P., & Nerlich, B. (2005). Disease metaphors in new epidemics: The UK media framing of the 2003 SARS epidemic. *Social Science & Medicine*, 60, 2629–2639.

9. Camus, A (1947) *La Peste*. Translated by Robin Buss. London: Penguin.

10. https://theconversation.com/coronavirus-if-we-are-in-a-war-against-covid-19-then-we-need-to-know-where-the-enemy-is-135274.

11. https://www.rt.com/uk/519300-breathing-is-offensive-weapon/.

12. Honigsbaum, M. (2020) *The Pandemic Century: A History of Global Contagion from the Spanish Flu to Covid-19*. London: Allen, p. 11.

13. Dodworth, L. (2021) *A State of Fear: How the UK government weaponised fear during the Covid-19 pandemic*. London: Pinter & Martin, Chap. 4.

14. This was a scheme whereby employees were paid a percentage of their normal wages to stay at home.
15. *DAILY MAIL (London)*, 23 March, 2020.
16. *Daily Telegraph*, 9 April 2020.
17. *The Express*, 13 March 2020.
18. *The Daily Telegraph (London)*, 16 March 2020.
19. *MailOnline*, 30 April 2020.
20. *MailOnline* 2 April 2020.
21. *The People*, 7 February 2021.
22. Thibodeau, P. H & Boroditsky, L. (2011) 'Metaphors we think with: the role of metaphor in reasoning'. *PloS ONE* 6(2): e16782.
23. The counting of metaphors is a fraught activity for metaphor scholars who usually come up with different results, for example whether a phrase of 2 words (e.g. 'biological war') is counted as 2 metaphors or just one metaphor). In my own view it is one metaphor.
24. An excellent overview of mixed metaphor is given in Gibbs, R. W. (ed.) (2016) *Mixing Metaphor*. Amsterdam: John Benjamins.
25. Charteris-Black, J. (2012). Shattering the bell jar: metaphor, gender and depression. *Metaphor & Symbol* 27: 199–216.
    Charteris-Black J. (2016). 'The 'dull roar' and the 'burning barbed wire pantyhose; Complex metaphor in accounts of chronic pain'. In R. W. Gibbs (ed.) *Mixing Metaphor*. Amsterdam: Benjamins. pp. 155–178.
26. https://www.bbc.co.uk/news/health-52124554.   Accessed   29 March 2021.
27. https://headtopics.com/uk/six-coronavirus-patients-describe-their-ordeals-with-the-disease-11796271. Accessed 29 March 2021.
28. https://www.bbc.co.uk/news/uk-52353275. Accessed 29 March 2021.
29. https://news.sky.com/story/coronavirus-this-is-how-it-feels-to-be-in-intensive-care-with-covid-19-a-survivors-graphic-story-11973549. Accessed 29 March 2021.
30. *MailOnline*, 1 October 2020.
31. *The Guardian*, 30 April 2020.

3

Metaphors of the Pandemic: Fire and Force of Nature

The Fire Frame

Outside of science fiction, war is viewed as a definitively human crisis, however, since the virus partly originated in natural disruption it seemed equally relevant to draw on frames for disaster originating in the natural world. In this chapter I discuss the fire frame—words such as 'ignite', 'blaze' or 'fan the flames'—and the 'force of nature' frame—words such as 'overwhelm', 'surge' and 'turn the tide'. A virus is at the margins of life and can also be viewed as not alive: in the hinterland of life, it challenges the boundaries of categories. As with war metaphors, the fire frame offered a readily available means for understanding the seriousness of the situation and provided a framework for understanding epidemiology and the contagious nature of the disease; some researchers (e.g. Semino, 2021[1]) have suggested this was an especially effective frame for public health communication purposes.

A typical example of this is:

And Dr Jonathan D Quick, former chair of the Global Health Council…told the Guardian: "The best case is that the Chinese *conflagration*

© The Author(s), under exclusive license to Springer Nature Switzerland AG 2021
J. Charteris-Black, *Metaphors of Coronavirus*,
https://doi.org/10.1007/978-3-030-85106-4_3

is brought under control, the smaller '*flames*' we've seen *flare up* in other countries are *extinguished*, there's little or no spread to new countries or continents, and the epidemic *dies out*.[2]

Here the speaker is rhetorically drawing on knowledge of forest fires to urge caution, since it is known that even a small flame can unexpectedly reignite a fire. So, the biology of the pandemic is modelled by knowledge of the dynamic nature of forest fires. There was nothing essentially novel about the fire frame, The Australian virologist Frank MacFarlane Burnet studied conditions in the overcrowded barracks of American recruits where the Spanish flu originated in 1918 and argued that it was "intimately related to war conditions"; these young American recruits who came to Spain and then transferred to France came into contact with men from many other nations and created the conditions for the Spanish flu pandemic: "If the early American epidemics supplied the initial spark for the pandemic we can be certain that it was fanned into a flame in Europe".[3]

In his retrospective account, Defoe had framed the spread of the plague in 1665 as analogous to the spread of fire in London the following year:

> It seemed enough that all the remedies of that kind had been used till they were found fruitless, and that the plague spread itself with an irresistible fury; so that as the fire the succeeding year spread itself, and burned with such violence that the citizens, in despair, gave over their endeavours to extinguish it, so in the plague it came at last to such violence that the people sat still looking at one another, and seemed quite abandoned to despair; whole streets seemed to be desolated, and not to be shut up only, but to be emptied of their inhabitants; doors were left open, windows stood shattering with the wind in empty houses for want of people to shut them.

Even though the Great Fire of London is believed to have contributed significantly to the ending of the plague, the intensity of the destructiveness and the range of spread of the two disasters was equivalent. Fire and illness have a long association in human experience, with their shared embodied experience of heat (fever) and the use of fire in sterilisation. I have argued that fire is a primary domain of experience for our under-standing of how embodied phenomena are transmitted, or 'spread'.[4] Fire has served as a frame for the pandemic in a way that is similar to war: both are metonyms for disaster. As with a virus, the speed of fire's spread can be encouraged by careless human behaviour. It may be that war and fire metaphors are similar because they trigger a more general 'disaster' frame and both activate the moral frame of Care and Harm. In her blog *Metaphors in the time of coronavirus*,[5] Nerlich classifies 'floods', 'storms' and fire-related terms under the general category of 'Disaster Metaphors' but for me, 'war' could equally be considered a 'disaster', albeit one that is man-made.

An examination of the press demonstrates the extensive use of the expression 'forest fire' by medical experts to raise the level of urgency regarding the crisis and so heighten the need for action:

A "concerning" number of mystery Covid-19 cases in New South Wales is "akin to a *smouldering forest fire*" that could suddenly *flare up*, an epidemi-ologist has said.[6]

"Yet again, the UK has been slow to act, delaying decisive action until the last moment," said Dr Stephen Griffin, an associate professor at Leeds University's School of Medicine. "Much *like a forest fire, the longer things burn, the harder they are to extinguish*, and the more *damage ensues from both the fire and the water*. Ironically, by delaying, the harm done to industries and society will be far worse compared to had the advice of Sage been fol-lowed in September."[7]

Dr Julian Tang, an honorary associate professor in the department of respi-ratory sciences at the University of Leicester, told MailOnline: '…Unless you stop people from travelling this is going to continue to happen. 'It's *like a forest fire*. If you don't have *major fire breaks all along the forest line* you're going to get it *jumping across to other parts*, unless you *make a fire break around the whole forest boundary*. If you shut down just one part the virus goes around it so it's going to be, I suspect, that this half-term lock-down may happen.'[8]

In these cases, the experts are explaining the conditions and process by which a virus may spread with reference to the fire frame as part of an argument to introduce control measures; in the months prior to the pandemic viewers all over the world had seen horrifying images of the bush fires in Australia, and in California, so the situation invited the fire frame as it was already cognitively active among global audiences. But fire metaphors were not simply to scare, but to advocate political responses such as a Lockdown: one does not simply ignore a fire. However, it was not the immediate situation alone that triggered the fire frame; the forest fire as a way of modelling both the extent and intensity of the spread of disease had been around for much longer. As Defoe comments:

> ...when I say that the violence of the distemper, when it came to its extremity, was like the fire the next year. The fire, which consumed what the plague could not touch, defied all the application of remedies; the fire-engines were broken, the buckets thrown away, and the power of man was baffled and brought to an end.

The time when he was writing of course predated the science of epidemiology and the only explanations that Defoe could offer were inauspicious sightings of Comets. For Defoe both fire and war provided relevant frames:

> So the Plague defied all medicines; the very physicians were seized with it, with their preservative in their mouths; and men went about prescribing to others and telling them what to do till the tokens were upon them, and they dropped down dead, destroyed by that very enemy they directed others to oppose.

As with coronavirus, the virus had no respect for medical training or knowledge. In other cases, fire metaphors were used in press headlines to highlight rhetorical evaluation such as representing politicians in the heroic role of firemen:

> Sunak still *firefighting* coronavirus *flames*.[9]

One of the emotional reactions triggered by the pandemic was panic buying of essentials such as toilet paper, UHT milk, medicines and pasta, and this socially disruptive behaviour that offended the moral frame of Fairness and Cheating, was also framed as a fire with cause and effect relationships expressed by the 'spark' metaphor:

> CORONAVIRUS has *sparked* panic with members of the public rushing to buy hand sanitiser from shops across the country.[10]

> Coronavirus panic buying *sparks vicious fight* between shoppers over toilet rolls;

> Supermarkets draw up emergency plans to 'feed the nation' if coronavirus causes mass shutdown—amid fears panic-buying could *spark food riots* and empty shelves.[11]

Here the serious problem of stockpiling contributing to shortages is profiled with the fire frame, the idea being that once a process has begun it has the potential to spread exponentially. We see similar emotional senses modelled on the concept THE CAUSE OF AN EMOTION IS THE CAUSE OF A FIRE:

> Supermarkets across the country have struggled to keep up with demands for goods such as toilet paper, hand sanitisers and soap due to panic buying *ignited by* the global coronavirus crisis.[12]

> Trump *fans flames* of Chinese lab coronavirus theory during daily briefing.[13]

> 'Awful' test and trace *sparks* fury as threat of local coronavirus '*flare ups*' intensifies.[14]

In each case the author relies on a fire-related word to prime the reader for an emotional response. This representation of emotions carries with it the implication that the emotions aroused are likely to be intense ones, based on the concept THE LEVEL OF INTENSITY OF AN EMOTION IS THE LEVEL AND INTENSITY OF A FIRE that derives from the Fairness and Cheating moral frame.[15] Evidently the pandemic caused such disruption that emotions were likely to run high and motivated acts of accusation and blaming as to the cause of the outbreak, which Trump attributed to China. He viewed this argument as crucial to his chances of being re-elected, since if China had caused the outbreak, this would deflect from his own incompetence in handling the pandemic as the US was soon topping international comparison tables for coronavirus fatalities. The 'China Virus' accusation combined appeals to the moral frames of Fairness and Cheating and Loyalty and Betrayal. In so far as China denied the accusation it also appealed to Honesty and Dishonesty.

Metaphors highlighted the various stages and progressions of the pandemic, and implied that they were following the natural cycle of fire. They could either focus on cause, response or end point—both fires and pandemics might burn themselves out when deprived of fuel. The highlighting of fire as a process that had an organic cycle was effective in providing re-assurance that the pandemic would eventually end and could be influenced by human interventions through, for example, the creation of 'firewalls'. As well as triggering negative social reactions, the risk of an onset of Covid-19 was also referred to as a 'spark', many employed this metaphor as a warning about the return of the disease:

> Public health authorities have warned, however, an increase in human interaction to massage economic activity could *spark a* 'second wave' of infections.[16]

> Wuhan launches mass coronavirus testing project after new cases *spark* second wave fears; Wuhan, China, where the coronavirus first emerged, has had a string of new cases that have *sparked* fears of a second wave of Covid-19.[17]

> Second wave begins: Huge spike in cases *sparks* panic at COVID-19 hotspot; FEARS of a second wave of coronavirus has erupted after South Korea reported a spike in cases in the country.[18]

Once it had become established the simile 'like a fire' was used 43 times and 'like a wildfire' was used 18 times in the British press in the 1-year period from 1st March 2020:

We're thinking about Covid-19 the wrong way. It's not a 'wave'—it's a wildfire; *like a fire*, the virus relentlessly seeks out its *fuel*, humans, and will keep *spreading* as long as it has access to that[19]

'It is *like a fire spreading*,' New York Governor Andrew Cuomo, of the alarming spread of the virus from the New York City epicenter. '*The fire*, it doesn't max out in one place, but it *consumes* where it is and it's *moving out*.'[20]

However, some used 'like a fire' to argue for particular responses to the pandemic. In the following, the forest fire analogy is part of an argument *against* active intervention:

Pandemics tend to grow exponentially to begin with, then to peak and *burn out—like a fire that starts in a dry forest and uses up all the fuel*. A pandemic will recede even if humans don't intervene, in other words, because the bug that causes them either kills those it infects or leaves them more or less immune.[21]

One of the rhetorical purposes of fire metaphors was to caution against certain behaviours as being likely to increase the rate of infection; a metaphor that was commonly used here was 'add fuel to', as in:

Meanwhile, Andrew Hayward, professor of infectious disease epidemiology at University College London, said that mixing at Christmas would *add "fuel to the fire"* of a respiratory infection peak in January.[22]

People were earlier warned not to *add "fuel to the fire"* by mixing in groups, as almost half of all major hospital trusts in England deal with more Covid-19 patients than at the peak of the first wave of the virus.[23]

The metaphor usually commented negatively on some aspect of Covid-19 related behaviour. Such cautionary metaphors were sometimes developed to explain objectively and reflect on Covid-19 policies:

Pakistan's government has also hailed its smart-lockdown system of local-
ised shutdowns which avoided a lengthy national hibernation. ...Dr Sultan
said despite the promising signs, he remained cautious.

"At the end of the day I keep reminding people that this is *like smouldering
embers* and the *embers* are there. You provide them with *fuel* and with a
little bit of *oxygen*, they will *flare up*," he said...[24]

'Until you really *extinguish* (coronavirus) with a vaccine or treatment, there
is always that risk of a *flare up*. We have to be very careful and think over
the long term,' Kashkari said.[25]

Explanatory, or heuristic metaphors such as these were effective in
enhancing general public understanding of epidemiological principles.
The speaker here is employing the fire frame to explain the process
through which infection takes place; the virus behaves in the way that fire
behaves and because fire is a much more tangible and known entity
than coronavirus it provides an effective heuristic for understanding the
process by which viruses spread. It is quite neutral in that there is no criticism implied of social actors or their policies.

But in other persuasive genres such as opinion articles, the fire frame
was employed differently: to argue either in favour of, or against, specific
policies. These are the predicative purposes of metaphor because they
assign particular attributes to actors. The 'fanning the flames' metaphor
implied a higher degree of intentionality and blame than simply 'adding
fuel' because it implies more effort and to greater effect. This is the case
in the following criticism of the Scottish government for its tardiness in
introducing testing in care homes:

However, a policy for mandatory testing of all new care home residents was
not announced by the Scottish government until April 21. Mr Leonard
said: "Ms Freeman has serious questions to answer as to why she claimed
that the vast majority of untested discharged patients were sent to their
own homes. The impact of coronavirus in Scotland's care homes has been
little short of horrifying and it is clear that discharging infected patients to
care homes has played a key role in *fanning the flames* of this virus."[26]

These hyperbolic metaphors express moral outrage with the incompetence of actors: the return of infected patients to care homes was a major scandal throughout the UK. In the following article the 'fanning the flames' metaphor is used to morally condemn the 'neo-liberal' or non-interventionist responses to the pandemic by arguing that they were causing unnecessary damage:

> The strategy proposed in the Great Barrington declaration—a letter signed by an international group of scientists—is the latest salvo in an ongoing battle of ideas for how to tackle the pandemic. It calls on governments around the world to abandon strategies that suppress the virus until we can better cope—through working test-and-trace programmes, new treatments, vaccines and more—for the radically different approach....

> William Hanage, a professor of epidemiology at Harvard, likens the strategy to protecting antiques in *a house fire* by putting them all in one room, standing guard with *a fire extinguisher* but simultaneously *fanning the flames*.

> "If the *blaze* outside the room were adequately controlled then maybe, just maybe, they would be able to stamp out all the *embers*," he said. "But this approach is to actively encourage the *fire*. The risk is that too many *sparks* make it through and all you're left with is *ashes*."[27]

Professor Hanage argues that it is counter-productive to simultaneously 'cocoon' vulnerable groups such as the elderly without also controlling the virus 'outside the room'. It introduces the arsonist frame of intentional damage and implies that libertarians and supporters of the Great Barrington declaration are on the margin of criminality. An even more vivid image for condemning policies viewed as likely to increase infection is the metaphor of 'pouring petrol' on a fire. It has an even higher Speech Act force because it not only involves an action like 'fanning' but also premeditation and planning to obtain the petrol, and hence criminality (arson). In a much-quoted phrase:

> Nicola Sturgeon has appeared to rule out reducing Covid restrictions in Edinburgh this year by comparing a shift to Level 2 to *"pouring petrol on smouldering embers.*[28]

The metaphor construes this as a deliberate act to increase harm. Others used the metaphor to criticise policies relating to schools:

> Scott Pughsley, a teacher in Preston, last night likened the reopening of all schools next month to '*pouring petrol on the smouldering embers of a fire* to make it go boom and keep *burning*'.[29]

The 'pouring petrol' metaphor is one that assigns the attribute of deliberate incompetence to political actors. These metaphors are different from the heuristic explanatory metaphors we looked at previously because predicative metaphors assign blame to political actors by arguing that their policies are deliberately incompetent and dangerous. This is how it is used in the context of reporting the anti-vaccine movement:

> While not championing every bizarre conspiracy, Wakefield has been happy *to pour petrol on the flames* and take credit for the movement's growth.[30]

Reflecting the interests of its elderly readership, the *Daily Mail* took a consistent and forceful line of opposition to opponents of the Covid-19 vaccine. They linked them to their progenitor, Andrew Wakefield, who had been responsible for raising suspicions about the MMR vaccination leading to the resurgence of measles. Fire metaphors could therefore be used to condemn libertarians and their policies because they actively and intentionally promoted harmful practices by encouraging vaccine hesitancy, but they could also be used to condemn anti-libertarians as in the following:

> Into this debate, Professor Neil Ferguson has apparently once again sought *to pour petrol on* the proverbial *fire*. He has suggested that 20,000 deaths could have been saved if we had gone into lockdown a week earlier.[31]

The report is keen to undermine the moral credibility of someone who is opposed to libertarian policies and supported an earlier lockdown by emphasizing the inaccuracy of his previous predictions:

Readers will remember we last heard from Ferguson when he resigned from the Scientific Advisory Group for Emergencies (SAGE) because he was breaking lockdown rules to conduct an affair with a married woman. This is the same scientist who presented claims, which were not peer reviewed, to suggest 500,000 people would die of coronavirus. In 2002 he predicted that up to 50,000 people would likely die from mad cow disease but there were only 177 deaths from BSE. In 2005, Ferguson predicted that up to 150 million people could be killed from bird flu but only 282 people died worldwide.

The main thrust of the article is to defend government policy and metaphor is employed to undermine the moral credibility and professional competence of anyone who criticised this policy. The moral frame that is appealed to here appears to be one rejected by the social intuition model: honesty and dishonesty. The author claims that Ferguson is dishonest because he has a record of fabricating the facts and they use a fire metaphor to emphasise this claim.

Empirical Research & Analysis

From the start of the pandemic the British press made extensive use of metaphors from the lexical field for fire in stories on the theme of coronavirus; this includes 'firewall', 'spark', 'ignite', 'flare up', 'burn', 'blaze', 'flame', 'conflagration', 'extinguish', 'embers' and 'ashes'.[32] A sample identified on the Nexis database for reports classified by the theme of 'Coronavirus' for the period from February 2020 to February 2021 is shown in Table 3.1:

Table 3.1 The lexical field of fire in the British Press (2020–2021) (number of stories containing the 'fire' term)

	2020								2021	
	Feb	Mar	April	May	June	Oct	Nov	Dec	Jan	Feb
Flare up	15	74	175	353	428	132	122	60	88	74
Spark	593	2412	2385	2421	2237	1832	1627	1548	1910	1614
Extinguish	28	47	95	54	54	53	59	46	40	45
Total	636	2533	2655	2828	2719	2017	1808	1654	2038	1733

Use of the fire lexicon rapidly increased in March through to June and then declined, followed by a rise again (after a quiet summer) during the second wave, especially in January 2021. The pattern is similar to that of war metaphors, which supports the argument that they both originate from a more general 'disaster' frame.

In the empirical research measuring beliefs about pandemic behaviour, respondents to the online survey were asked to read the short story below that includes 8 fire metaphors (words or phrases) and I will refer to as the 'fire vignette'. Metaphors are shown here in italics, but the version used in the research did not indicate the metaphors. The vignette is approximately the same length as the previous vignettes (90–100 words):

Fire Vignette

Imagine it is 16 March 2020, 3 months after the *sparks* of Coronavirus *ignited* in China. Italy is *burnt* badly as *the blaze spreads* across Europe. In the UK, Prime Minister Boris Johnson *fights the fires* by *dispatching a brigade* of retired and newly qualified healthcare workers to *tackle the conflagration*. 251 new cases have been reported today and as the nation's death toll reaches 35. While Cheltenham races were given the go ahead, Johnson now calls for *the creation of a firewall* by instructing non-key workers to work from home and advising the public to avoid pubs and restaurants.

As previously, I asked respondents to rank five statements relating to their personal decisions in order of their importance from high importance to low importance. The personal decisions were based on various aspects of government guidance and were as follows:

1. Carry on life as normal.
2. Go out as normal but begin 2 m social distancing everywhere.
3. Limit outings to 1 hour a day for essential trips and exercise only.
4. Strictly limit outings to essential trips only.
5. Put their household into complete quarantine.

A total of 78 respondents completed the fire vignette and findings are shown in Table 3.2:

Table 3.2 Responses to the fire vignette

Behaviours	1st rank	2nd rank	3rd rank	4th rank	5th rank
Carry on life as normal	1	0	0	4	73
Go out as normal but begin 2 M social distancing everywhere	4	2	30	40	2
Limit outings to 1 hour a day, for essential trips and exercise only	16	38	22	2	0
Strictly limit outings to essential trips only	42	27	8	1	0
Put their household into complete quarantine	15	11	18	31	3

When comparing these results with those for both the war vignette (Table 2.2) and the literal vignette (Table 2.3) there were no statistically significant differences between responses either when compared with the literal vignette or the war vignette again supporting the view that there is little impact of metaphor on personal decisions about current lived experience and if there is an impact of metaphors it is not one that people are necessarily aware of. However, some comments supported the view that 'fire' metaphors do have some influence by activating a more general frame for 'disasters' that is rooted in an evolutionary need to avoid causes of harm:

The statement that includes language relating to fire is by far the most powerful and terrifying statement.

The metaphors referring to fires and blazes invoked a sense of urgency. The fire version almost feels as though there is a sense of "too late"-ness and serious actions need to be taken straight away.

The one describing the fire raging is horrifying, and creates a much more vivid picture of the destructive quality of the pandemic.

"Fire" (version B) seems quite effective as it relates to real-life events which have been experienced in the past and which are much easier to understand than a pandemic.

Here respondents' reactions reflect the moral frame of Care and Harm that is triggered by the fire frame. Respondents seem generally more favourable to the fire frame than to the war frame even though it did not appear to influence the importance they placed on behavioural responses. The extent of the danger presented by the virus imposes a moral obligation on governments to respond quickly and effectively. Some governments, such as those in South Korea and Germany, responded much more effectively than others such as the United Kingdom. Analysis of the fire frame therefore provides insight into how beliefs about moral frames such as Care and Harm are aroused by metaphors, even though it does not necessarily influence behaviour.

The Force of Nature Frame

A wide range of metaphors represented the pandemic as a force of nature: increases in the number of people affected were routinely described as 'surges', while health systems that could not cope were described as being 'overwhelmed' as a 'tsunami' of patients arrived for treatment. Many of these metaphors involved the movement of vast amounts of water but I am using a more inclusive term 'force of nature' to include verbs that refer to experience of the force of nature such as 'overwhelm', 'batter' and 'strike' that also include the effects of extreme weather. Rather than simply 'catching' coronavirus, national leaders were 'struck down' while their economies were 'battered', each hoping somehow to 'turn the tide' on the pandemic. In this frame, as with the war and fire frames, there was a rhetorical onus for those in charge of health policy to emphasise the extent and gravity of the crisis by framing its effect as a force of nature that had the potential to cause disasters, which we have seen was also the case with the 'war' and 'fire' frames.

While 'war' metaphors and some 'fire' metaphors framed the crisis as man-made, the force of nature frame construed coronavirus as caused by non-human, 'objective' forces to which governments and societies needed urgently to respond. Metaphors contributed to this rhetorical goal; consider the metaphors in the following for example:

London hospitals are facing a "continuous *tsunami*" of coronavirus patients and some are likely to be *overwhelmed* in a few days, according to Chris Hopson, the chief executive of NHS Providers—which represents hospital bosses… Speaking to BBC Radio 4's Today programme, he said: "They are *struggling* with the *explosion* of demand in seriously ill patients. They are saying it's the number arriving and *the speed* with which they are arriving and how ill they are. They talk about *wave after wave after wave*. The words that are used to me are that it's a continuous *tsunami*. As one said to me, it's much bigger and large numbers with a greater degree of stretch than you can ever have possibly imagined. The CEOs are concerned that all that extra capacity is now being used up very, very quickly. We've got the *surge* capacity at the ExCel centre but this is filling up very quickly."[33]

Here the speaker, who was responsible for the capacity of hospitals in London to treat Coronavirus patients, had the rhetorical imperative of making people aware of the extent of the crisis and the speed with which it was developing, for this purpose he relied heaving on metaphors such as 'tsunami', 'overwhelmed', 'surge' etc. He was not alone, in New York:

Mayor Bill de Blasio on Wednesday warned that four million people in New York City will get coronavirus after *attacking* Donald Trump's 'false hope' of lifting the lockdown at Easter and *slamming* Mitch McConnell for '*blocking*' funding.… Labeling the coronavirus pandemic 'a growing crisis and growing challenge' he told New Yorkers to 'not *let their guard down*'. Doctors in the city have described an '*apocalyptic*' *surge* in patients in *overwhelmed* hospitals.[34]

The physical force verbs in the first sentence frame the verbal actions of Mayor Bill de Blasio and Donald Trump as a boxing bout. Words such as 'overwhelmed' and 'surge' in the second sentence refer to the numbers of people who had contracted the disease. While the first sentence concerns human agents, the second is about non-human ones, but what both share is emphasising the physicality of embodied experience. Leaders never just 'caught' coronavirus in the way that they caught a cold, but were typically 'struck down' by it:

UK Prime Minister Boris Johnson, US Senator Rand Paul and even Charles, Prince of Wales are just some of the world leaders who have been *struck down* by the coronavirus.[35]

The UK's Brexit negotiator David Frost has all been *struck down* with coronavirus, while Scottish Secretary Alister Jack has also quarantined after noticing symptoms.[36]

Another cabinet minister has been *struck down* by coronavirus-type symptoms following Prime Minister Boris Johnson and his Health Secretary Matt Hancock.[37]

Over the year there were 579 reports that referred to someone as being 'struck down with' or 'struck down by' coronavirus. As with words like 'tsunami' or 'surge', there was the idea that they were affected by a physical force; here the metaphor was not describing the number of patients but the *severity* of the effect of the disease on a person's health. Just as if they were a boxer receiving an upper cut to the jaw they were 'floored by' the disease:

Fit and healthy 40-year-old '*floored*' by coronavirus begs people to stay indoors.[38]

Speaking live from her home in York on today's Good Morning Britain, Dawn explained that she was self-isolating after being "*floored*" by illness.[39]

There are of course different ways of describing such metaphors, we could consider coronavirus as a physically powerful opponent, but the metaphors seem to highlight the impact on patient(s) rather than the agency of the disease. So, for example, if we compare the active and passive use of 'overwhelm', there were 165 stories over the year that featured the phrase 'overwhelmed by coronavirus' whereas there were only 24 reports over the same period that employed an active form of 'overwhelm' ('overwhelms', 'overwhelming', or 'overwhelmed'). A comparison of passive and active forms is shown in the following examples:

Passive Form:

Furious Tory rebels DEMAND Michael Gove publish his evidence after he claims the NHS—including Nightingale emergency hospitals—could be '*overwhelmed*' by coronavirus cases without the Government's tier system.[40]

Ski towns and luxury retreats report rising number of cases amid concern hospitals could be *overwhelmed by* coronavirus patients.[41]

Active Form:

More than 75 per cent of Britons need to socially isolate for the attempt to stop coronavirus *overwhelming* the NHS.

Collapse in cancer treatment as coronavirus *overwhelming* hospitals.[42]

This preference for the passive is because the main topic of the story is the entity that is affected by coronavirus, 'Nightingale hospitals' and 'ski towns' in the above examples, so the passive voice facilitates this topicalization of the affected entity rather than the agent.

We find a similar pattern with other physical force verbs such as 'batter', over the same period 104 reports included the passive form 'battered by coronavirus' or 'battered by Covid-19' whereas there were only 36 stories that include the active form 'coronavirus/Covid-19 batters' and 'coronavirus/Covid-19 is battering':

Passive Form:It called for the leftover funds instead to be reinvested in support for local economies *battered by* coronavirus.[43]

Spanish tourism is being *battered by* a coronavirus 'tsunami' with 'no new bookings' at some hotels as the disease spreads in the country, a leading hotels body has claimed.[44]

Active Form:The board's plaintive message is echoing across many of the poorest parts of the Madrid region as the second wave of coronavirus *batters* Spain and once again threatens to overwhelm the health system in and around the capital.[45]

CORONAVIRUS has '*battered*' the travel industry in recent months and the cruise sector in particular.[46]

Though there was also a tendency to transform 'batter' into a compound adjective with 58 reports with 'Covid-19/coronavirus-battered':

The plight of Bowser and other renters on the edge foreshadows a national crisis that's expected to grow next year, with states and cities that granted renters a reprieve amid the *coronavirus-battered* economy now wrestling with what comes next.[47]

While I haven't been reduced to daytime pyjamas, I know that looking better will improve my *coronavirus-battered* morale.[48]

The adjectival use of 'battered' highlights the effect on the victim ('economy' and 'morale') rather than on the agent ('coronavirus'). As a form of 'invisible enemy', it was not easy for journalists to construct an image schema for the active role of the virus: it was more evident what it *did to* people, or to social entities such as the economy, and so the dominant topic of most reports was the *effect* of the disease—whether on individuals or society generally—rather than providing a detailed explanation of the biological processes by which individuals contracted it.

Two much used, and hence rather tired metaphors from the force of nature field were 'wave' and 'tsunami'; the phrase 'tsunami of' was used in 9872 reports and typically it was in contexts such as 'tsunami of cases' (77) and 'tsunami of coronavirus' (41) as in:

Relaxing coronavirus restrictions over Christmas could lead to an "unrelenting *tsunami*" of cases, the head of the Royal College of Nursing has said.[49]

The Royal College of Nursing warned the NHS faces an "unrelenting *tsunami*" of coronavirus this winter.[50]

There could be a 'tsunami of' just about any negative social phenomenon that was attributed to coronavirus including 'job losses', 'eviction', 'vaccine misinformation', 'mental health problems' etc. so that the metaphor had become so conventional it became a synonym for 'large amount'. At times, it also became a form of institutional 'get out of jail card' through which businesses could blame any changes they desired (for reasons of profit) on the pandemic. Many businesses indicated they would no longer send hard copies of letters 'because of the pandemic'—without any suggestion that their real motivation was to save on postage costs. Dishonesty was not the sole prerogative of politicians but widely practiced by those seeking to gain commercially from the pandemic.

Another 'force of nature' metaphor that was commonly used to describe the economic impact of Lockdowns was 'body blow':

Bosses across England have demanded VAT and tax relief be extended throughout 2021 after a third lockdown announcement delivered a '*a body blow*' for thousands of firms—which face a 'cliff edge' as support ends in the spring.[51]

The second national lockdown is a "*real body blow*" for business, the director-general of the Confederation of British Industry (CBI) has said.[52]

Sometimes it was a specific aspect of economic policy that was described as a 'body blow':

Rishi Sunak's decision to extend the furlough to October is *a body blow* and we should all be fearful[53]

Backtracking on the reintroduction of crowds is *a body blow* for sport;[54]

Typically, this force of nature metaphor was used in direct quotation of a business representative who was keen to use hyperbole to attract attention to the specific area of economic activity that he or she felt was negatively affected by Lockdown related policies. For example, on the announcement of the second Lockdown Chamber of British Industry boss Carolyn Fairbairn said: "This is a real *body blow*, firms have worked very hard to become Covid-safe". Physical force metaphors are common in descriptions of the economy and market trading as in expressions such as 'a bout of' and could be considered as related to boxing or wrestling, but since they really describe the impact of some external abstract event (e.g. unemployment) as if it were exerting a physical force on the body I include them within the 'force of nature' field because there is very little impression that people who are experiencing Lockdowns can do anything about them, they become rather like the weather, an irresistible, necessary but somewhat oppressive external force.

It became formulaic to consider the increases in the number of cases as if they were 'waves' so that there appeared to be a relentless series of 'waves of infection'; these were enumerated as 'the first wave', the 'second wave' etc. and at the time of writing the Prime Minister is warning that a 'third 'wave' may soon be washing into the United Kingdom from Europe. These are summarised in Table 3.3:

It is a well-established practice to refer to a series of pandemic infections as 'waves', this is because, when represented on a graph, the patterns of increase and decrease 'rise' and 'fall' in spatial terms, and so they appear like waves on the surface of the sea. But the conventional metaphor also carries notions of irresistibility and inevitability. There is a focus on the phenomena itself as a *natural force* rather than one caused by *human* agency. All one can do is, like a surfer on his board looking out to the mid horizon to catch the big surf, be prepared when the big wave comes and then perhaps stay on its surface rather than be crushed under it. In the overall frame of things, a 'wave' is less frightening that a 'tsunami' which, is course, a type of wave that by definition 'overwhelms' all in its path. The 'wave' metaphor was typically used to express a degree of fatalism about the pandemic, and at times the literal sense could be reactivated as a way of extending the metaphor, for example when a 'third wave' was developing on mainland Europe, Boris Johnson warned:

> Yesterday Boris Johnson told MPs it was "inevitable" the third wave would reach the UK, but insisted the country was prepared. Earlier in the week he said publicly it was likely to *"wash up on our shores"*[55]

He had used a similar metaphor in relation to the second wave the previous July:

> He told Sky News: 'I am worried about a second wave. You can see a *second wave* starting to *roll across* Europe. We have to do everything we can to prevent it reaching these shores.[56]

Table 3.3 'Wave' in British newspaper coronavirus reports (Feb 2020–Feb 2021)

First wave	8326
Second wave	>10,000
Third wave	1689
Fourth wave	106
Fifth wave	8
Sixth wave	1

The metaphor is a type of reification, as if it were possible to prevent a material entity—like a boat of asylum seekers–from arriving. Of course, the 'waves' metaphor had become a familiar trope in relation to illegal immigration with the phrase 'waves of migrants':

> THE dire economic impact of the global coronavirus pandemic is likely to propel new *waves* of migrants and refugees towards the richer parts of the world, the head of the Red Cross warned yesterday.[57]

Generally, in nationalist rhetoric, the container of Britain was in constant danger of being perforated or overwhelmed by foreign menaces of one form or another and the pandemic provided an opportunity for the restoration of Britain as a fortress or impregnable container.[58] Of course, the reality was somewhat different as it appears that the UK Border Agency agency was so ineffective it had not been able to return a single migrant to mainland Europe after Britain's departure in December 2020. In general, the collocations of 'waves' were negative ones, for example in a large corpus there were 'waves of': 'infections'; 'outbreaks'; 'protests'; 'illness'; 'layoffs'; 'droughts;' 'migrants'; 'lockdowns' and 'contagion' and 'grief';[59] there were also 'heat waves' and 'shock waves'. As with many liquid-based metaphors, they arouse powerful human emotions, typically fear.

Empirical Research & Analysis

As might be expected from the previous analysis of 'war' and 'fire' metaphors, 'force of nature' metaphors fluctuated with the disease itself; this is evident from Table 3.4 that shows the frequency of this lexical field with a rise in March and April 2020 followed by a decline in May and then an increase as the 'second wave' 'hit' in October 2020.

Table 3.4 shows us that the lexical field for the force of nature includes a number of nouns such as 'tsunami' and 'wave' related to the quantity and motion of seawater, but also several verbs related to force such as 'strike' and 'batter' (I searched for these verbs within 5 words of 'coronavirus'). 'Body blow' did not occur at all in the month prior to the onset

Table 3.4 Force of nature lexical field in the British Press (2020–2021)

	2020 (number of stories)								2021	
	Feb	Mar	April	May	June	Oct	Nov	Dec	Jan	Feb
Strike W5/ coronavirus	833	3691	4172	3527	3012	2903	2644	2365	2609	2152
Wave	343	2288	3946	4246	4093	5431	3917	3382	3754	2708
Overwhelm W5/ coronavirus	268	3152	3133	2288	1281	1675	1563	1457	2073	967
Batter W5[a]/ coronavirus	86	426	472	427	327	417	382	321	346	325
Tsunami	13	323	185	175	166	143	80	121	111	54
Trickle	20	132	170	172	139	85	195	56	107	61
Turn the tide	6	237	233	89	74	114	87	121	127	90
Body blow	0	26	29	35	23	36	83	30	28	24
Total	382	3006	4563	4717	4495	5809	4362	3710	4127	2937

[a]'W5' indicates that the 2 words occurred within a range of 5 words of each other

of Covid-19, and accelerated to more than double the previous month in October 2020, in the lead-up to the announcement of the second Lockdown on 31st October 2020, usually in the context of business leaders lobbying against Lockdown. Other words referred more generally to the actions of nature when it is experienced as exerting a massive force on the human body or on some aspect of the social system (health services, economy etc.). I have suggested that these verbs are metaphors because they all have a more basic primary sense of one entity impacting with force on another entity, as in 'hit', 'batter', 'overwhelm' and 'strike'. Typically, a tsunami would 'hit', for example:

> 'We are going into a war zone' NHS nurse warns coronavirus *'tsunami' to hit* Britain;[60]

> The coronavirus outbreak forced communities that were hardest *hit by the tsunami* to cancel or postpone memorial services, with some setting up altars for people to lay flowers.[61]

As with 'battered', 'hit' could also be compressed into a compound adjective:

> …horrifying scenes a *coronavirus-hit* aged care home in Melbourne[62]

Apart from the traditional grammatical analysis I have illustrated above (active versus passive voice), these physical force verbs can also be modelled with reference to the force dynamic approach.[63] This is an approach in which there is a role difference between two entities that are exerting forces. One force-exerting entity—the antagonist—(force A in Fig. 3.1) is considered for the effect that it has on the second force entity—the agonist—that tries to resist the force of the first entity (force B in Fig. 3.1).[64] The focal force entity is the agonist, and the antagonist force is the subject of verbs such as 'overwhelm', 'strike', 'hit' or deliver a 'body blow'; in the examples above 'coronavirus' is in the antagonist role while 'Britain, 'communities' and 'care home' are in the agonist role. These relations are summarised in Fig. 3.1

The two force entities act upon each other with the agonist either giving way to, or resisting, the force of the antagonist in their struggle over the human body or the health services that are affected by coronavirus. The body's immune system can be viewed as the agonist and Coronavirus can be viewed as the antagonist. The agonist resists infection either through its antibodies, or at the institutional level, medical services (force B), while the antagonist (coronavirus, force A) has an extrinsic tendency to put force on the body or on the medical services. When the force of the immune system is equal to the force of the antagonist (B=A), a stable state of health is maintained in the body. But when the antagonist overcomes the forces of resistance (antibodies) of the agonist (A > B), the body experiences illness as its equilibrium is lost. Whatever happens at the level of multiple individual bodies also governs what happens to medical services: there is equilibrium when their force in resisting the disease is equal to the force of the Covid-19 antagonist (A = B). Slogans like 'Protect the NHS'' can be viewed as increasing force B and contributing to social equilibrium. The model can be classed as 'causative', because it explains causes such as how a mass disease has the potential for medical services to be 'overwhelmed'. The force dynamic approach is especially appropriate in relation to health because it explains the relationship between internal agents—viruses—and resistance within the human body and the external health system.

Another force of nature metaphor that this theory accounts for is when leaders seek to 'turn the tide' on the virus:

FORCE A

ANTAGONIST:
Coronavirus and its capacity to infect

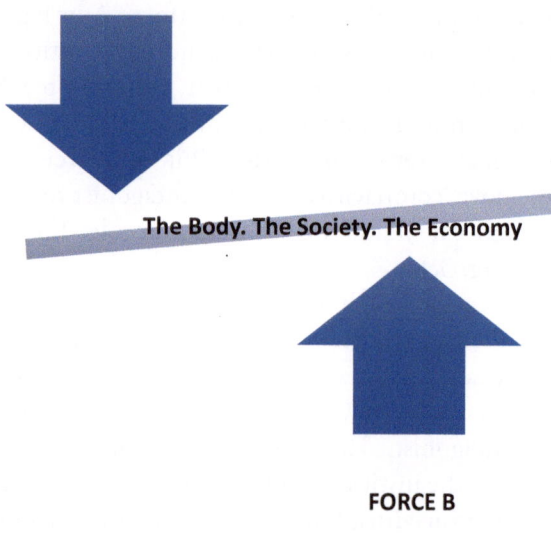

FORCE B

AGONIST:
The body's immune system / institutional resistance to disease

Fig. 3.1 Force dynamic model for Covid-19

'I believe that a combination of the measures that we're asking the public to take and better testing, scientific progress, will enable us to get on top of it within the next twelve weeks and *turn the tide*'.

Now I cannot stand here and tell you that by the end of June that we will be on the downward slope. …But what I can say is that this is going to be finite, we will *turn the tide*, and I can see how to do it within the next 12 weeks.[65]

As cases rose exponentially his claim to be able 'to turn the tide' became increasingly Canute-like. But Boris Johnson returned to the same metaphor later in the year, this time by personifying the virus and introducing a crime frame:

And that is how and why we are now beginning to *turn the tide*. If this virus were a *physical assailant*, an unexpected and *invisible mugger*, which I can tell you from personal experience it is, then this is the moment when we have begun together *to wrestle it to the floor*.[66]

Perhaps one of the reasons was to dispel the apparently ridiculous image of trying to reverse a force of nature. The 'mugger' frame legitimated a more robust response by the agonist: if the virus is a criminal, a mugger, then we have a warrant to lock him up and throw away the key! It also personalises his own strength in overcoming the mugger. He returned to his earlier claim in May:

In the darkness of March, I said that with hard work, we could *turn the tide* within three months. We have now passed through the peak. I said, if we could get an antibody test showing whether you have had the disease, it would be a huge step forward. Public Health England has now approved an antibody test which is 100 per cent accurate.[67]

After this Johnson preferred to forget the 'turning the tide' metaphor although the press returned to his '12-weeks' claim in a somewhat mocking tone:

"I just don't want to let people run away with the idea that this development is a home run, a slam dunk, a shot to the back of the net, yet. There's a long way I am afraid before we have got this thing beaten." Mr Johnson's cautious approach was in contrast to a press conference early on in the first wave of the pandemic, when he suggested that Britain could "*turn the tide*" against the outbreak of the coronavirus within 12 weeks.[68]

Boris Johnson is due to make a statement to the Commons tomorrow (Tuesday). He will be desperate to rally the nation. But that must be getting harder. All the way back in March he claimed that Britain could "*turn the tide*" in just "12 weeks". Unfortunately, tides have a habit of coming back in.[69]

In each case the journalist activates the force of nature frame to caution Boris Johnson for his initial over-optimism in being able to 'turn the tide' on the virus in 12 weeks when it became increasingly clear that government policy was always playing catch-up with the virus rather than taking the initiative by, for example, closing the borders. However, economy with the truth has been something of a hallmark of Boris Johnson and the 'turn the tide' metaphor was a double-edged sword: it invited feelings of hope but when these hopes were frustrated it appeared a hollow attempt to resist an irresistible force of nature.

Another metaphor of resistance into which the force-dynamic approach offers insight is the concept of '*surge-testing*'. A surge is a powerful natural force, as in the concept of a 'tidal surge'. We have one of these in the Bristol area known as the Severn Bore when surfers go out to enjoy the power of nature at the spring tides. As a Covid-related metaphor it was first used in July 2020 to signify a new concept:

> The US Department of Health and Human Services said it was adding short-term 'surge testing' sites in three metropolitan areas in Florida, Louisiana and Texas.[70]

It gradually took on the meaning of introducing testing in areas where there had been a surge in increases of positive cases of coronavirus:

> Nursing homes in these communities would only need to undergo 'surge' testing, done every three to seven days, if a new infection was identified.[71]

> Where is '*surge testing*' in the UK? So far, two cases have even found in Surrey, but testing is also expected to take place door-to-door in London, Kent, Hertfordshire and Walsall…*Surge testing* will see residents in the Goldsworth Park and St Johns area of Woking, Surrey, visited and requested to take a PCR test regardless of whether or not they are showing symptoms, while Egham is expected to be added to the list in coming days.[72]

The BBC offered an explanation of the concept and its purpose:

Surge testing is the roll-out of additional community testing of people who do not have any coronavirus symptoms. It aims to help scientists and public health officials learn more about the mutated Covid-19 variant found in Bristol and South Gloucestershire. It will also help reduce the spread of infection by finding asymptomatic cases and prompting people to self-isolate.[73]

The metaphor takes its primary sense from electrics where *'surge testing'* means testing an electrical system for an unexpected increase in voltage; so, it derives from electricity and carries the same objective scientific epistemology based on understanding cause-effect relationships:[74]

Surge tests are critical because they are the only test that finds turn-to-turn insulation weaknesses. These weaknesses start at voltages above the operating voltage of the motor and are precursors to serious failures and shutdown of a motor. Surge tests are also used to find hard shorts and a number of other mistakes in windings and coils.[75]

Even non-electricians can, hopefully, appreciate that a 'surge test' is an important safety procedure. Attraction of the metaphor is that *'surge testing'* appears to strengthen force B that of the agonist in strengthening its capacity to exert a counter force against Force A—the antagonist and to ensure balanced health in the society. As a concept it is oriented towards a social, institutional response rather than one that focuses on the individual body, although the two are, of course, interdependent.

In the survey respondents were asked to read the following vignette and then to rank possible responses by their order of importance as with the previous vignettes:

Force of Nature Vignette

Imagine it is 16 March 2020, 3 months after the *wave* of Coronavirus *struck* in China. Italy is *drowning* as the *tsunami sweeps* across Europe. In the UK, Prime Minister Boris Johnson *sends out the lifeboats* by *pressganging fleets* of retired healthcare workers for a search and rescue operation. 251 new cases have been reported today and as the nation's death toll reaches

35. While Cheltenham races were given the go ahead, Johnson now calls for *survival mode*, instructing non-key workers to work from home and advising the public to avoid pubs and restaurants.

The results are shown in Table 3.5:

The results are not significantly different for any of the behaviours from those for the 'literal', 'war' or 'fire' vignettes; however, there is a difference from the literal vignette as regards the percentage of people that rank first the most secure, or most risk-sensitive action 'Put their household into complete quarantine'. For the literal vignette only 12.7% ranked this as the most important, whereas with the force of nature vignette 23.2% ranked the response first, nearly double the percentage for the literal vignette. This compared with 28% for the war vignette and 19.2% for the fire vignette. The similarity of the ranking of responses for the different metaphor vignettes provides support for the view that they derive their influence from a common 'disaster frame'-irrespective of whether these disasters have 'human' or 'natural' causation. Metaphors, whether in war, fire or force of nature vignettes, all heighten an awareness of the dangers of coronavirus by activating a generic disaster frame that is rooted in evolutionary survival instincts and the powerful moral emotion of avoiding Harm. There was some support for this interpretation in the comments:

I think the more decorative the language, the more visual and real the situation feels. When the language is colder and more detached the situation doesn't feel as real, it's easier to detach from the situation somehow.

Table 3.5 Responses to the force of nature frame

Behaviours	1st rank	2nd rank	3rd rank	4th rank	5th rank
Carry on life as normal	2	0	1	3	63
Go out as normal but begin 2M social distancing everywhere	2	5	29	33	0
Limit outings to 1 hour a day, for essential trips and exercise only	16	31	17	4	1
Strictly limit outings to essential trips only	33	25	8	3	0
Put their household into complete quarantine	16	8	14	26	5

Respondents also commented on the potential of fire to arouse an emotional response that made them critical of government policy:

> Some of the accounts portray a calmer message than the others and felt more 'factual'. Some accounts felt fearful and used more dramatic language. These more fearful accounts made me feel like I wanted the government and the public to take stronger action!

While the influence of metaphor induced frames is not always one of which we are fully conscious, there is sufficient evidence from the qualitative component of the research of the potential for metaphor to influence behaviour during a pandemic.

Notes

1. Semino, E. (2021). "Not Soldiers but Fire-fighters"—Metaphors and Covid-19. *Health Communication*, *36* (1), 50–58.
2. *Daily Star Online*, 1 March 2020.
3. Burnet, F. M. & Clark, E. (1942). *Influenza: A Survey of the Last fifty Years. Monograph from the Walter and Eliza Hall Institute of Research in Pathology and Medicine*, no 4. Melbourne: Macmillan. In Honigsbaum, M. (2020) *The Pandemic Century: A History of Global Contagion from the Spanish Flu to Covid-19*. London: Allen, p. 35.
4. Charteris-Black, J. (2017a) *Fire Metaphors: discourses of awe and authority*. London & New York: Bloomsbury. pp. 19–26.
5. https://blogs.nottingham.ac.uk/makingsciencepublic/2020/03/17/metaphors-in-the-time-of-coronavirus/.
6. *The Guardian (London)*, 28 December 2020.
7. *The Independent—Daily Edition*, 1 November 2020.
8. *MailOnline*, 18 September 2020.
9. *The Sunday Times (London)*, 28 February 2021.
10. *Express Online*, 3 March 2020.
11. *MailOnline*, 3 March 2020.
12. *mirror.co.uk*, 10 March 2020.
13. *The Guardian (London)*, 16 April 2020.
14. *Express Online*, 12 June 2020.

15. Charteris-Black (2017a), *Fire Metaphors: discourses of awe and authority.* London & New York: Bloomsbury, p. 55.
16. *MailOnline*, 28 April 2020.
17. *Daily Star Online*, 18 May 2020.
18. *Express Online*, 8 June 2020.
19. *The Guardian*, 4 August 2020.
20. *MailOnline*, 4 April 2020.
21. *The Sunday Times (London)*, 1 March 2020.
22. *telegraph.co.uk*, 19 November 2020.
23. *Express Online*, 31 December 2020.
24. *telegraph.co.uk*, 20 August 2020.
25. *MailOnline*, 14 April 2020.
26. *The Times (London)*, 25 May 2020.
27. *The Guardian (London)*, 7 October 2020.
28. *telegraph.co.uk*, 14 December 2020.
29. *MailOnline*, 21 February 2021.
30. *DAILY MAIL*, 17 July 2020.
31. *The Express*, 11 June 2020.
32. See Charteris-Black, J. (2017a) *Fire Metaphors: discourses of awe and authority.* London & New York: Bloomsbury, pp. 28–32 for a full account of the lexical and semantic fields for fire.
33. *The Guardian*, 26 March 2020.
34. *MailOnline*, 25 March 2020.
35. *MailOnline*, 27 March 2020.
36. *Express Online*, 30 March 2020.
37. *MailOnline*, 28 March 2020.
38. *Daily Star Online*, 24 March 2020.
39. *mirror.co.uk*, 26 March 2020.
40. *MailOnline*, 29 November 2020.
41. *The Guardian (London)*, 4 April 2020.
42. *The Sunday Telegraph (London)*, 10 January 2021.
43. *The Independent (United Kingdom)*, 3 August 2020.
44. *MailOnline*, 12 March 2020.
45. *The Guardian (London)*, 18 September 2020.
46. *Express Online*, 31 March 2020.
47. *The Independent (United Kingdom)*, 17 December 2020.
48. *MailOnline*, 20 July 2020.
49. *telegraph.co.uk*, 18 December 2020.

50. *The Independent—Daily Edition*, 19 December 2020.
51. *Mail Online*, 5 January 2021.
52. *i-Independent Print Ltd*, 2 November 2020.
53. *MailOnline*, 13 May 2020.
54. *telegraph.co.uk*, 31 July 2020.
55. *telegraph.co.uk*, 24 March 2021.
56. *MailOnline*, 30 July 2020.
57. *The Daily Telegraph*, 25 July 2020.
58. See Charteris-Black, J. (2006) 'Britain as a Container: Immigration Metaphors in the 2005 Election Campaign'. *Discourse & Society* 17(6), 563–582.
59. https://www.english-corpora.org/corona/.
60. *Express Online*, 25 March 2020.
61. *The Guardian (London)*, 11 March 2020.
62. *The Guardian (London)*, 15 August 2020.
63. See Charteris-Black, J. (2017a) *Fire Metaphors: discourses of awe and authority*. London & New York: Bloomsbury, pp. 55–61.
64. Talmy, L. (1988) Force Dynamics in Language and Cognition. *Cognitive Science*, 12(1), pp. 49–100.
65. *MailOnline*, 19 March 2020.
66. Boris Johnson Coronavirus Speech 27 April 2020.
67. *MailOnline*, 16 May 2020.
68. *The Times (London)*, 10 November 2020.
69. *telegraph.co.uk*, 21 September 2020.
70. *Express Online*, 7 July 2020.
71. *MailOnline*, 9 September 2020.
72. *Express Online*, 1 February 2021.
73. https://www.bbc.co.uk/news/uk-england-bristol-55947013.
74. In the next chapter I will discuss how the metaphor 'circuit breaker' also derived from electricity.
75. https://electrominst.com/test-technology/surge-tests/?cli_action= 1616436477.033.

4

The Pandemic as Zombie Apocalypse

Introduction

This chapter explores how fantasy provided frames for articulating a present in which humanity appeared to be threatened with destruction; these frames derived from science fiction films and dystopic fiction on topics such as environmental destruction and other apocalyptic themes. While there had been pandemics before, in the West the last one was over 100 years previously. In terms of the breadth and depth of the crisis the closest analogy was with the Second World War—and even this was not a good analogy as the pandemic did not originate from political decisions, although contrasting attitudes to mask-wearing reflected conflicting political ideologies. For those outside of the health sector, and other key sectors of the economy, the requirement to stay at home permitted more time for rumination: there was now permission to fantasise, introspect and reflect on the meaning of life. Given the time now available for staring out of the window, playing computer games and doom-scrolling,[1] it is perhaps not surprising that science fiction based fantasies provided the themes for such reverie. With the outbreak of mutations, the virus itself proved to be something of a Shape Shifter and was soon offered a

© The Author(s), under exclusive license to Springer Nature Switzerland AG 2021
J. Charteris-Black, *Metaphors of Coronavirus*,
https://doi.org/10.1007/978-3-030-85106-4_4

leading role in dystopic reflection. As the world gradually stopped, there was also time for moral reflection and an intuition grew among some that it was actually, we, humanity, who were the virus. Film-watching and fantasy-based allegories framed the pandemic as a viral invasion that might lead to a zombie apocalypse. In a world where some of the living had died, and the life of many of those still living took on a death-like stillness, science fiction metaphors offered a framework for articulating existential uncertainty and exploring moral possibility. As the worlds of science and science fiction converged in lived experience, some drew on the familiar trope of the zombie apocalypse when they wanted to interpret the strangeness of this surreal world and created memes such as 'We are the virus' as a form of allegorical comment.

In the first part of this chapter, I explore the fantasy of a zombie apocalypse as articulated in the British press and on Twitter and in the second part I suggest that moral intuitions related to feelings of disgust about man's role in causing the pandemic manifested themselves in allegories about the Sanctity of Nature and were expressed by the "We are the virus" meme. It was man's activities that had degraded the planet and created the conditions in which the virus, like a zombie, could emerge. In the broader context of the climate change crisis, the 'We are the virus' meme found the same imaginative seedbed as zombie apocalypse narratives: both offered a theme in which moral retribution was nature's way of settling scores. If we had been fairer in our treatment of the planet, we would not now be suffering the consequences of trying to cheat the laws of nature. In the discourse of coronavirus there was, at the allegorical level, a quest to avoid becoming one of the living dead by re-engaging with nature and this reflected the more internal psychological experience of Lockdown.

Moral psychology assists in interpreting such metaphor frames and allegories and, as we saw in Chap. 1, Jonathan Haidt proposes six moral foundations of which Sanctity and Degradation is one. Metaphors and allegories that invoke this moral frame provided an alternative to the dominant discourse of Care and Harm that was mainly expressed in literal language. Apparently trivial housekeeping decisions such as whether or not to visit a relative, to wear a mask, to go to the shops in person or whether or not to have a kick around in the park were construed in terms of moral decision making—and much public communication in the pandemic appealed on the basis of taking care of loved ones and avoiding harming strangers. But the imagination also required a larger more encompassing moral narrative, an allegory, and it is this gap that was filled by the Zombie Apocalypse frame and the 'We are the virus' memes.

The Zombie Apocalypse Frame

There were many newspaper reports on the topic of Coronavirus that included a reference to zombies: a total of 1066 news reports in the UK national press over a one-year period from 1st March 2020 made reference to 'zombie'. *The Express Online* was the most common among these, featuring 'zombie' in 147 of their reports during the year. In these, the onset of the pandemic bore resemblance to the scenario of a zombie apocalypse in which zombies, devoid of cognition, were spreading inexorably through infection, breaking up the bonds of society and demanding new modes of survival as a response. There was also evidence of the frame on Twitter:

> The current Big Brother Germany cast doesn't know about COVID-19. In 2008, Black Mirror's Charlie Brooker created Dead Set, a TV show (in Netflix) where the Big Brother cast doesn't know about a zombie apocalypse. THIS MAN'S MIND". + link to Dead Set.[2] (86 comments, 1600 retweets and 9000 likes)

Some of the comments recalled *Dead Set* or indicated that they were re-watching it. Another introduced the frame in relation to panic shopping:

> One expert likened #coronavirus to panic buying to coping with a zombie apocalypse: 'You can do what you can. It might not make a lot of sense, but it provides a feeling of at least doing somethin'. + link to article in the LA Times.[3] (24 comments, 80 retweets and 282 likes)

Another subscriber, motivated by the desire to discourage panic buying, offered comfort with the reassuring message that this wasn't in fact a zombie apocalypse:

I don't know who needs to hear this, but panic buying is a feedback loop.
Shortage of supply
Fear of lack of supply
The power and water grids aren't going down.
Farm and foods supply chains aren't shutting down.
Covid-19 isn't a zombie apocalypse.[4]

(24 comments, 78 retweets and 444 likes)

Some were associated with the 'prepper' genre: people who were making preparations to survive an apocalypse. Surviving a zombie outbreak is more feasible than surviving a takeover by Artificial Intelligence as zombies are slow moving and *lack* intelligence.

If Covid-19 has taught us anything, it's that the world is completely unprepared for a zombie apocalypse.[5] (78 comments, 178 retweets and 1000 likes)

After all these years waiting for the zombie apocalypse to happen, you think we would have been better prepared for #Covid-19. + link to a black and white image of a zombie.[6] (30 comments, 86 retweets and 312 likes)

The prepper theme was also evident in the British press and there was a report on a study to identify the cities that offered the best chance of surviving a zombie apocalypse and a map showed the best place to be in UK in this event:

Highlight: A ZOMBIE APOCALYSE may not be on the cards any time soon—or so we hope—but scientists have now revealed the best place to live if the dead were to rise up.

In the event of a societal collapse, such as a zombie apocalypse, researchers believe the best place to be would be somewhere which already has an environmentally friendly and sustainable infrastructure in place. For that reason, energy firm Save On Energy has been ranking the most sustainable cities in the UK, which would also be best suited for a zombie apocalypse ....
"But if zombies were to take over, how prepared would your city be?

Our zombie survival index sought to find out which cities are least prepared for a zombie apocalypse based on each of the eight different factors: solar energy produced per year, farming area, the number of farmers per city, air quality, outdoor space, recycling centres, wind farms, and the number of electric-vehicle charging points.[7]

I was surprised to find that Oxford came up as the city *least* likely to survive a zombie apocalypse, though not surprised to find that Derby was, apparently, the third least likely to *survive* such an event. As when during the pandemic it became a skill to know which supermarket would be stocking toilet rolls and where to buy flour, surviving a zombie attack required knowledge and survival skills. But why else was the experience of the pandemic understood with reference to surviving a 'zombie apocalypse'? The cause of pre-modern pandemics was typically understood with reference to some form of divine retribution, sometimes accompanied by a visible sign. In Defoe's *Journal of the Plague Year,* he refers several times to a comet that was visible prior to the plague's arrival in London, and suggested an association between the two. But post-enlightenment humanity in most parts of the world does not give much credence to the predictive capacity of comets. However, people do watch movies and the zombie genre has grown exponentially over the last 20 years to the extent that there are at least 500 zombie films. The powerful narrative of the living dead is itself a trope for a consumerist culture: as mankind stumbles towards extinction through over-consumption of resources, there is torpor in the response. But since zombies, being slow moving, are quite easily shot they present a more manageable vision of survival than do other forms of destruction—for example a meteor strike or global flooding. The scenario of a climate change catastrophe by the flooding of coastal cities would cause much greater disruption than a zombie attack.

With the threat of extinction, it is not surprising that we need an additional trope for death other than that offered by personifications such as the Grim Reaper, or the Four Horsemen of the Apocalypse. Both these personifications did occur with 'the grim reaper' featuring in 297 reports (over 20% up on the previous year) and 302 times in the Coronavirus Corpus[8,9] and 'the four horsemen' occurring in 143 reports (10% up on the previous year) and 76 times in the Coronavirus Corpus. But both these personifications were supernatural beings whereas zombies were part of nature, and originally one of us—even one of our own family or loved ones who had become infected—and therefore served as a persuasive metaphor for the man-made environmental crisis. The changes in human habits that have forced wild animals into greater proximity with humans have created the perfect conditions for viruses to transfer from one to the other; once coronavirus had infected one person that person could then go on to infect many others, following the rigid laws of epidemiology. The inevitability of this process and the apparent lack of human agency once the infection had set in made the zombie apocalypse a trope for explaining how the infection spread, how it could be responded to, and for dealing with some of the anxieties arising from the pandemic. At least the zombie came from the world of science fiction and allowed us to contemplate destruction in a way that *might* still be avoided, just as when we leave the cinema, we leave behind some of our anxieties. The zombie, then, became a personification of the coronavirus victim, suddenly the infected individuals, even though they might be our loved ones, had lost agency and could be the causes of our own infection. The zombie hazmat suit became a popular fancy-dress outfit that took the pandemic into the realm of fun and fantasy.

Another related question we may ask ourselves is why 'zombie' metaphors were more frequent than vampire ones during the pandemic? In the Coronavirus Corpus there were 2098 instances of 'zombie' but only 651 instances of 'vampire'.[10] This was because zombies fitted in visually with the strange appearance that many cities around the world had taken on as they emptied of people, so the focus was less on the zombies themselves than on the outcome of a zombie attack—streets that were emptied as all their inhabitants had either fled or been infected or consumed by zombies. A number of reports commented on the strangeness of the appearance of emptied places:

> Meanwhile, former cabinet minister Damian Green has called on civil service workers to "set an example" and return to Westminster, which he said now looks like a "zombie apocalypse".[11]

> Zombie outbreak: THIS is how a zombie apocalypse would look based on coronavirus pandemic; CORONAVIRUS has forced streets to empty and the majority of people to stay inside with scenes reminiscent of zombie

apocalypse movie, and now one expert has revealed what an outbreak of the living dead might look like.[12]

It seemed that the zombie apocalypse frame was the one that most readily available, the word 'apocalypse' occurred 2106 times in the Coronavirus Corpus—similar to that of 'zombie'.[13] On hearing accounts of the pandemic, the wife of a Canadian diplomat, Michael Kovrig, who had been jailed in China on espionage charges since 2018 said he was:

> astonished to learn about the details of the COVID-19 pandemic and remarked that it all sounded like some *zombie apocalypse* movie.[14]

It was the zombie movie that came to mind rather than the vampire movie. The vampire was really a trope for the exploration of sexual fantasies, but these were largely absent from pandemic discourse, it was not sexy seeing the incapacitated bodies of poor victims of the disease being physically rotated at regular intervals. Similarly, social distancing hardly encouraged close physical relationships, except within 'bubbles', and for those enjoying online dating, it was again likely to be through remote forms of contact. By contrast, the bodies of patients suffering from Covid-19 had taken on some zombie-like qualities: they were highly infectious, they needed to be isolated and the agency of the individual had apparently been taken over by the virus. In intensive care units some patients resembled the living dead as the damage to their organs was so great that, though partially alive, part of them had died. Recovering Covid patients walked slowly with their heads slumped a bit like zombies. The physical resemblance of coronavirus victims to zombies contributed to the 'zombie' frame. There were a few references to 'zombie virus' and a game that referred to this was removed from a platform in China:

> A video game where players shoot "selfish zombies" infected with coronavirus has been removed from the Steam gaming platform in mainland China. The Coronavirus Attack game, which remains available to download through Steam in other countries, involves firing an "anti-zombie" weapon at infected characters trying to escape the country.

"Selfish-zombies virus has infected throughout the country. The Virus carriers are attempting to flee the country," the game's description states. "Your purpose is to prevent the selfish zombie virus carriers from escaping and infecting the world. You must destroy the carriers as much as possible and collect more DNA to develop more lethal trait properties and clear the carriers before they develop corresponding immunity."[15]

Perhaps the Chinese authorities were concerned that the 'zombie virus' concept might lead to the mistreatment of those thought to be carrying the disease from Wuhan and who were selfishly trying to escape the city by concealing their symptoms. Concern about this behaviour, and the role of the zombie frame in condemning it, is analysed in a study of posts made to the Chinese microblogging site Weibo in the last week of January 2020. The authors identified posts that expressed the collective fear towards Wuhan escapees:

Really wrecking the country and ruining the people. Die in their own house if they want! Do not run around! Really behaving like zombies, biting people everywhere. (translated from Chinese)

The eight cases in Sichuan and four cases, now, in Xian were all brought by them. Are they behaving like zombies? Not only may they have contracted a fatal disease, but they also intend to bite other people.[16] (translated from Chinese)

In Chinese culture a zombie is a reanimated corpse that feeds on not-yet-decayed human remains and their blood and so is closer to the western concept of a vampire. Escapees from Wuhan are viewed as dangerous 'zombies' because by trying to leave the city they are knowingly spreading the virus. Throughout history there have been instances of abuse and indeed execution of those thought to be carrying a lethal virus and this was the case in some non-western cultures where particular social or ethnic groups were associated with causing infection. For example, in India Muslims generally were blamed for spreading the virus after a large Muslim rally in New Delhi in March 2020 organised by the Islamic group Tablighi Jamaat. An Islamophobic hashtag #Coronajihad was exploited by right-wing Hindu nationalists to associate Muslims with the bioterrorist intention of deliberately spreading the virus among Hindus as a form of Jihad.[17] The hashtag was used more than 170,000 times in one week and contributed to a climate of religious intolerance towards Muslims who were seen as traitors. So, there were cultural variations in how the zombie frame was interpreted. While for western audiences the bodies of Covid-19 patients may have looked a bit like zombies in their loss of agency, in China they were employed, along with other animal metaphors, for the moral condemnation of the excessive individualism of those who were not observing the legal restrictions that had been placed on movement. By bringing attention to socially harmful behaviour, the zombie frame served as an enforcer of moral values. The Chinese zombie frame seems to integrate several moral frames: Harm, Cheating and Subversion (by breaking the rules), Betrayal and because of the inherently revolting behaviour of zombies, Degradation. By integrating all these moral frames, the zombie frame was likely to be highly persuasive to audiences. By contrast in India, the association made by extreme Hindu nationalists between a religious identity, Muslim, and the spread of coronavirus framed Muslims as infringing the moral frame of Loyalty

Other aspects of the zombie frame that were exploited by the press, and especially by the *Express Online*, were how to prepare a response to a major 'zombie' crisis. One article described how The US Centre for Disease Control and Prevention developed plans for how to respond to a zombie apocalypse scenario:

The CDC has, therefore, drafted a contingency plan explaining what to do if a zombie outbreak ever occurs. According to some scientists, the "zombification" of living beings already exists in nature and similar infections may even affect humans.

Rear Admiral Ali S, former director of the CDC's Office of Public Health Preparedness and Response, explained in 2011 the protocols the CDC has in place for a zombie outbreak. In a blog post titled Preparedness 101: Zombie Apocalypse, he said: "You may laugh now, but when it happens you'll be happy you read this, and hey, maybe you'll even learn a thing or two about how to prepare for a real emergency."

According to Dr Khan, the CDC will respond to a zombie outbreak much in the same way it responds to any disease or viral threat. He said: "If zombies did start roaming the streets, CDC would conduct an investigation much like any other disease outbreak. CDC would provide technical assistance to cities, states, or international partners dealing with a zombie infestation. This assistance might include consultation, lab testing and analysis, patient management and care, tracking of contacts, and infection control." Dr Khan has also outlined things people at home can do during the zombie apocalypse, such as preparing vital supplies to weather the storm.[18]

It is first worth noting that the zombification is represented as something real, part of nature, like coronavirus, and unlike vampires, contingency plans provide evidence of this (there are none for vampires). Part of the scenario of a real public danger is a rationale response, and the one described in the article reassured readers that there is a procedure in place to respond to a zombie outbreak, perhaps rather more so than there had been for a coronavirus outbreak. The idea of being overwhelmed by a numerous mass of individuals was something that the vampire trope did not really provide as they are lone operators, but zombies, though not organised, are everywhere.

Another, aspect of the zombie frame that motivated human-preparedness for the pandemic was the claim made by some specialists that it had motivated their original interest in epidemiology:

> Let's face it, viruses that cause "the sniffles" aren't what get most of us into virology. Some colleagues quote zombie apocalypse movies as inspiration for entering the field, and it's true that there's a certain macabre thrill in studying these terrible pathogens. But there are really only a few viruses able to kill us within days of infection.[19]

This suggests that it was the excitement of watching zombie films and perhaps the heroic roles they offered to zombie-slayers that encouraged people to research viruses: it took them into a world where their fantasies could indeed play out into reality. Other science fiction genres were also activated by the pandemic, indeed the marketing of a film called World War Z had to be modified to remove any reference to China as the source of a zombie virus:

Then there is the bleakly pertinent case of World War Z, whose script was amended at the insistence of Paramount executives to remove any reference to its zombie virus originating in China, as it did in the source novel by Max Brooks. In a recent interview, Brooks explained how crucial China had been to the story, because of the regime's capacity to cover up a virus's early spread.[20]

Although it is not yet known how the virus originated, Trump's 'China virus' epithet was designed to exploit the familiar frame from science fiction of an evil villain planning the disruption and eventual destruction of the west.

The 'zombie' frame also occurred frequently in the domain of financial reporting, as the genres of finance and economics are attracted to colourful metaphors that take on an allegorical role as in 'White Knights' for example, as they make concepts more accessible. Table 4.1 shows there were many references to 'zombie companies' and other 'zombie' compound nouns.

The Daily Telegraph offers a definition of the 'zombie firm':

In the last decade, that hasn't happened. Interest rates were slashed to just about zero, a 300-year low, and a couple of minor tweaks aside have just about stayed there ever since. The result? Lots of what economists started referring to as *"zombie" firms*, a term first coined when Japan slashed interest rates to zero in the Nineties. They are the living dead: not quite alive, but still staggering on anyway. There are lots of them out there. A report by KPMG last year estimated one in seven UK companies could effectively be *"zombies"*.[21]

Table 4.1 'Zombie' compound nouns in the British Press (1st March 2020–28th Feb 2021)

Zombie apocalypse	126
Zombie company(ies)	101
Zombie firm(s)	47
Zombie film(s)	21
Zombie outbreak(s)	17
Zombie economy	5
Zombie infection(s)	5
Zombie virus(es)	4
Zombie army	4

The author is perhaps a little ahead of the times as the earliest use of 'zombie companies' in the British press is:

> Mr Takenaka's reforms are expected to lead to the collapse of many of these so-called *"zombie"* companies. Yesterday Mr Okuda said that the failure of some of the largest firms among the walking corporate dead would be a sign that the government was serious this time about reform.[22]

The earliest use of 'zombie firms' was in March 2002:

> Banks' so-called bad-loan disposals have so far mainly involved booking higher loan-loss provisions in their accounts, which cuts into their capital but fails to remove the loans from their balance sheets or kill off *zombie firms*.[23]

In response to the pandemic crisis governments around the world sought to protect their economies by supporting businesses, but, according to the argument of financial reporters, these were fundamentally inefficient businesses and the implication of the metaphor 'zombie company' is that it is one that is not worth supporting as it is unlikely that the business will 'return from the dead':

> A lot of the money thrown at supporting workers was going to *zombie workers* at *zombie companies*.[24]

> Ordinarily, governments should avoid bailing out companies that would otherwise be unable to continue trading. When they do, the resulting entities are popularly known as *zombie companies*, meaning cash flow is insufficient to cover their interest expense.[25]

Sometimes these metaphors were extended to include a motion verb of walking:

> The response to the 2008 crisis, with low interest rates and almost free money, allowed a legion of zombie companies to keep *staggering* on.[26]

Rishi Sunak's scaled-back job support scheme will 'pull the rug' from under so-called '*zombie companies*' who have been *limping* along through the pandemic.[27]

The winding down of state support schemes will trigger an increase in corporate defaults and insolvencies. *Zombie companies* that have been *kept on life support* by taxpayer handouts will no longer be able *to stumble on*.[28]

The ailing condition of the company is described by the motion verb and draws on the image of zombies marching slowly with their bodies limp and lifeless, looking at the ground. In the original zombie film genre, in films such as *White Zombie*, zombies were depicted as sleepwalkers rather than flesh-eating monsters; this tradition only developed after *Night of the Living Dead* in 1968. These uses in the press seem to be activating the earlier schema of the sleepwalking zombie. There was also the use of metaphors from the survival of the fittest frame:

Zombie *firms* must be slain to save the strong[29]

And at the very heart of this *zombie economy* are the empty offices in towns and cities across the country, amid claims that working from home is not only viable for most white-collar workers, but somehow beneficial and more productive.[30]

Sometimes the 'zombie firm' metaphor was extended:

Alongside *zombie firms* are *zombie households*, a small but desperate demographic that took on more consumer debt to pay bills but have little hope of repaying it without a significant improvement to their fortunes.[31]

Here 'zombie firm' is extended to describe households that have no future prospects of returning to financial solvency after the crisis. The zombie frame was a way of criticising schemes like the furlough scheme and seems to argue for a return to a neo-liberal market driven economy and away from socialist concepts such as universal basic income that had preceded the pandemic. While, of course, it was only workers in businesses satisfying certain criteria who benefited from government subsidies, it seems that the metaphor was being employed as a way of reactivating old 'zombie' values.

We may question the extent to which the 'zombie firm/company' metaphor offers an allegory for the coronavirus pandemic; evidently the concept had been around throughout the twenty-first century, however, on searching March 2019–2020 I found that the frequency of the two terms was about half that of March 2020–2021 indicating that the metaphors were triggered by the pandemic context. Clearly, there were more businesses around that were in need of support during the pandemic but surely the authors of these reports could have used other language to express the idea of an unsuccessful company? So, there is some indication that the 'zombie apocalypse' frame including the visual state of empty streets, anxieties, and fears of attack etc. increased the use of the metaphor because it provided an allegory in financial reporting and economics. The allegory was that it was wrong for the government to 'prop up' companies that could not justify their own survival in a competitive market.

There was also a counter narrative on Twitter from those who were opposed to the vaccine; an account named MarceloBR2 tweeted:

#Globalists/ #VaccinePassports Understand, once and for all, it was never because of the #virus. All of this is purposeful, it is the globalist #Agenca of the #NewWorldOrder. They want a slave society, a society with the chip in their hands, a controlled society.

This was tweeted on 19th March 2021 under the hashtag 'zombie apocalypse' and has accompanying images related to vaccine passports that refer to the allegory of an embedded chip placed in the human body by Bill Gates; the frame incorporates the original zombie concept from Haiti that the loss of soul would create a braindead zombie who would comply with their bodies being used for labour. In this frame Haitian slaves were brainwashed with voodoo fears based on the terrible retribution of Baron Samedi to keep them from killing themselves. So, the dystopic vision offered by zombie narratives could be harnessed through allegory to the rhetorical goals of the anti-vaccine movement. Another tweet from an account NRC Canada depicted in black and white a street filled with silhouetted zombie-like figures and states that:

The view from our windows…It looks like the zombie #vaccine we have been working on isn't as effective as would have liked during initial testing. Be careful out there today!#zombieapolcalypse

It received 20 retweets and 43 likes probably because it provided a parody of the anti-vaccine movement.

Blending analysis offers some insights into how the zombie apocalypse became a familiar trope during the pandemic.[32] In this approach there are two input spaces corresponding with the two elements connected by metaphor but there is no linear direction that makes one of these prior to the other, so both input spaces are equally well known—this is appropriate in fantasy memes. Here it seems that conceptual knowledge of the input spaces for 'zombie apocalypse' and 'coronavirus pandemic' have sufficient commonalities in experience to then be accessed by a generic space that identifies what is shared between the input spaces and drives the blend. Both metaphors originate in some aspect of the natural world: in the case of the virus it is zoonotic proximity caused by man's influence on the environment, while in the case of the zombie it is natural infection, either, in the Hollywood tradition, by an animal bite or in the Haitian tradition from spirit control by a *boko* ('witch doctor') who could catch a soul in a vial and then use it to gain control over a man and turn him into a zombie who would then work for him. In either case there was loss of agency and the zombie frame clearly alluded to slavery. Both the 'zombie' and the 'pandemic' spaces demand some form of human response and appearance also motivates blends, so the restricted movement of walking in a hazmat suit makes the manner of walking resemble that of a zombie.

There are also some aspects of each input space that do *not* transfer to the blend, for example the magical forces of zombie culture in Haiti has numerous *iwas* or spirits such as Baron Samedi, a very powerful spirit dressed in black tails and wearing a black hat who is debauched, drinks, smokes and swears etc., this hardly transfers to the Coronavirus space, though there was a brief phase of videos going viral in which medical staff celebrated a patient survival with a dance.

Nurses are going viral as they spread positivity through song and dance in their daily fight against the virus. They have been dancing when a patient finally comes off a ventilator, breaking into song when COVID-19 patients are discharged, or TikToking in scrubs to boost positivity on the hospital floors. As a result, they are inspiring viewers all around the world.[33]

This event alludes to the general cultural idea of the dance of death rather than to Baron Samedi in particular. The pandemic has a role for government officials who give statistics and data which is rather removed from zombie culture, although there would presumably be the plotting of zombie sightings on maps. Nevertheless, there are sufficient commonalities to drive the blend and it is one in which there is potential for emergent space that predicts future developments. The blending analysis of 'coronavirus as zombie' is depicted in Fig. 4.1.

In the figure there are two input spaces: zombie apocalypse and the coronavirus pandemic, and under the influence of the generic space, common features such as the origins in the natural world, infection, loss of agency, social response and the physical appearance of the world are blended together from these inputs. They also have an emergent structure, so that for example there is the question of whether zombies and viruses are living or dead entities, and they both have the potential for evolution—either to develop intelligence (zombies) or mutant varieties (viruses).

Part of the therapeutic attraction of the zombie genre is that it offers a threat that is somehow manageable, zombies are not like robots, aliens or artificial intelligence that do not necessarily have any need for humanity and may therefore seek to dispense with humanity. Zombies feed off human bodies and without them would otherwise starve: rather like the virus, we know that it is not in their interest to wipe out humanity, in the emergent structure they therefore present an *acceptable form of imaginative risk assessment*. With the right preparedness we could just about survive a zombie attack and therefore the metaphor blend argues that we could do so with the current pandemic. Some stories highlight how a zombie attack is just another form of disease that requires a management strategy. In the *Express Online* story discussed earlier:

The CDC's primary goal would be to investigate the virus's source, its transmission routes and how readily it is spread. The CDC's scientists would then work towards synthesizing a cure, if possible, aided by other US federal agencies. Dr Khan has also outlined things people at home can do during the zombie apocalypse, such as preparing vital supplies to weather the storm...[34]

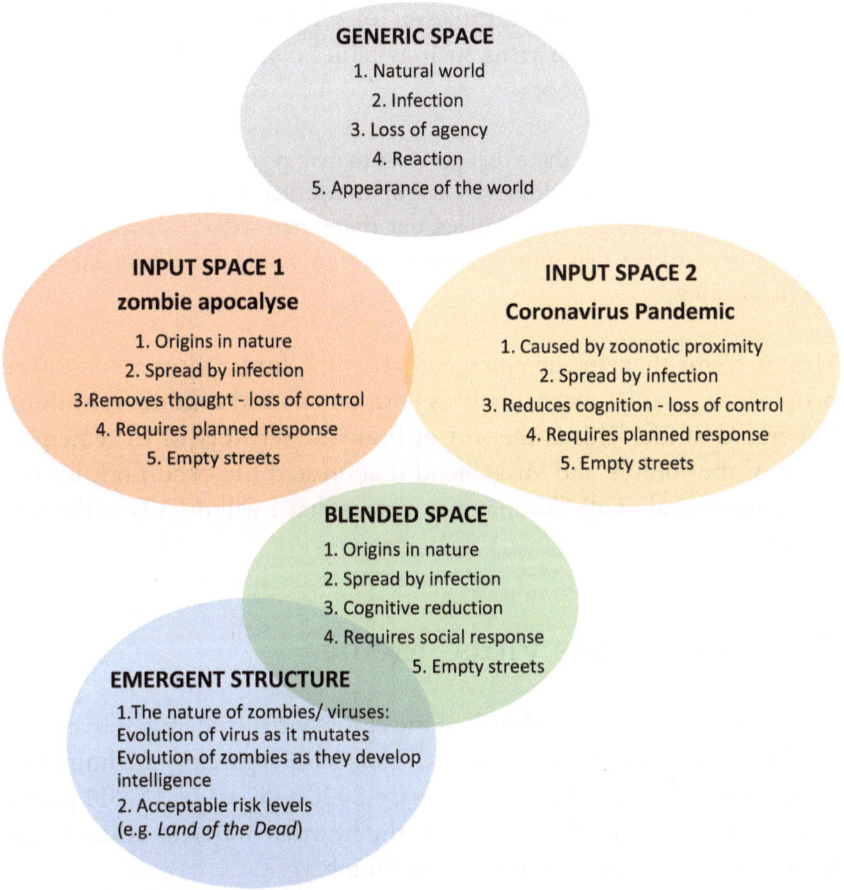

GENERIC SPACE

1. Natural world
2. Infection
3. Loss of agency
4. Reaction
5. Appearance of the world

INPUT SPACE 1

zombie apocalyse

1. Origins in nature
2. Spread by infection
3. Removes thought - loss of control
4. Requires planned response
5. Empty streets

INPUT SPACE 2

Coronavirus Pandemic

1. Caused by zoonotic proximity
2. Spread by infection
3. Reduces cognition - loss of control
4. Requires planned response
5. Empty streets

BLENDED SPACE

1. Origins in nature
2. Spread by infection
3. Cognitive reduction
4. Requires social response
5. Empty streets

EMERGENT STRUCTURE

1. The nature of zombies/ viruses:
Evolution of virus as it mutates
Evolution of zombies as they develop
intelligence
2. Acceptable risk levels
(e.g. *Land of the Dead*)

Fig. 4.1   Blending analysis of "coronavirus as zombie apocalypse"

The journalist is keen to emphasise the feasibility of dealing with a zombie apocalypse—just get down to the supermarket and fill up a large trolly of 'vital supplies' and if a zombie attack can be managed, how much easier a coronavirus infection? The discourse of reassurance was probably a comforting allegory for readers of the *Express Online*!

However, although currently manageable, the metaphor blend shown in Fig. 4.1 also has an emergent space in which just as zombies can develop intelligence, so the virus could mutate: in another *Express Online* article Dr. Ben Neuman, a professor of virology at the University of Reading, suggests that a virus such as rabies could evolve and conquer humanity. He told Yahoo:

> There are parasites out there that get close to making actual walking around zombies. But the real weirdoes locked up in Mother Nature's basement are the viruses. There are more viruses out there than we will probably ever discover and I bet that somewhere out there in nature something like this is happening.[35]

Here it seems that, in the emergent structure, future viruses could turn people into zombies, particularly as both viruses and zombies exist in the hinterland of life. This is the sort of futuristic territory of the emergent space of the zombie and virus blend that created the conditions for one of the most viral of all Coronavirus memes that I will discuss in the next section.

The "We Are the Virus" Meme

The background to the outbreak of the coronavirus epidemic was an existential angst throughout western democracies regarding an imminent environmental crisis. On 28th February 2020 a crowd of 15,000 people turned out in a rainy Bristol to hear the heartfelt warning of the young Swedish environmental activist Greta Thunberg:

> Our leaders behave like children so it falls to us to be the adults in the room. They are failing us but we will not back down. It should not be this way but we have to tell the uncomfortable truth. They sweep their mess under the rug and ask children to clean up for them. This emergency is being completely ignored by the politicians, the media and those in power. Basically, nothing is being done to halt this crisis despite all the beautiful words and promises from our elected officials. So what did you do during this crucial time? I will not be silenced when the world is on fire.[36]

In a topsy-turvy world the moral order had been turned upside down so that it was a child who was needing to explain to the world's leaders the true nature of what is, potentially, a *species* catastrophe—*our* species (amongst others). Once nations across the world had gone into Lockdown there was a conspicuous and rapid change in experience of the urban environment as the movement of people slowed down: airports slowed down to the rates they had been in the 1970s, commuter trains ran empty and traffic jams were replaced by the sight of fox and deer grazing on motorway sidings, or wild boar foraging on city streets, and goats coming into Welsh towns. From my balcony in Bristol the pollution haze that normally hangs over the city gradually dissolved and as the Lockdown continued so the layers of the Cotswolds became increasingly visible and the birdsong amplified, while at night the stars shone, and car lights twinkled on the distant horizon: yes, nature was reclaiming the city! This is the experiential backdrop that provided a frame into which, as attested by *The Guardian*, the "We are the virus" meme could take root:

> In the days, weeks and months after the world went into lockdown, we marvelled as animals began to venture out into the habitats we had deserted. Schools of fish were suddenly visible in Venice's cruise-ship-free waters. Flamingos flocked to Mumbai. A herd of fallow deer peacefully grazed on a London housing estate. Sheep visited a Locked-down Welsh MacDonald's. "WE are the virus," quickly became the most overused meme of the pandemic.[37]

It was the global nature of the meme that was emphasized in most reports:

> Cormorants are hunting fish in the now clear waters of Venice. Wild boars roam the avenues of Barcelona and wild goats the streets of Llandudno. Above Los Angeles are blue skies. From smogless Delhi, you can once more glimpse the Himalayas.
>
> "The Earth is healing, we are the virus," runs the meme spreading fast across the internet. It's a sentiment echoed by many policymakers, commentators and celebrities.[38]

The prototypical structure of social media posts took the form of an image of the new wondrous natural phenomenon, accompanied by a written comment (see figure 4.2). The image could be in diverse media including photography, film, graphics, cartoons or any mixture of these. So, for example, a close-up photograph of a bee collecting pollen from a flower could be accompanied by a link to a newspaper article reporting on the use of pesticides, an image of two pandas mating after a long period of infertility could be linked to a report on the regeneration of wildlife. A tweet from China that was 'liked' 954,200 times showed two elephants in Yunnan that had fallen over intoxicated after breaking out of a village compound and drinking 30kg of corn wine. But the darker side was also widely shared: posts, especially from India, depicted suffering or dead elephants: a photograph of a pregnant elephant that had died after eating plastic bags or junk food with a textual expression of moral outrage. As is often the case, those most widely circulated either evoked disgust or elicited the opposite emotion of awe for the beauty, or Sanctity, of nature.

The rhetorical purpose of such posts showed considerable variation. It could be to explain an aspect of environmental degradation with a view to modifying human behaviour; to display strong feelings of anger about human relationships with other species (perhaps therapeutic to the author); to pass moral judgement on a specific act of cruelty by a human agent towards another species or simply to celebrate the sanctity of nature by demonstrating its regenerative power (figure 4.2 shows three examples of tweets on this meme). But if nature was restoring itself and *we* are the virus, then, following the logic of this allegory, coronavirus was earth's vaccine, and it could restore nature to its pristine beauty.

Some observers noted that the argument of the meme was potentially an eco-fascist one. If people were welcoming, and even celebrating the potential of Coronavirus to eliminate mankind because this would ensure the survival of 'nature', then they were moving towards the same theories that had motivated searches for 'purity' throughout history: genocide has often been offered as a way of restoring the sanctity of the people. If mankind's impact on the environment was so deadly as to threaten its survival, then this could only be counterbalanced by the destruction of humanity regardless of suffering. In terms of natural justice, the elimination of humanity by a virus was the only solution that would enable the survival of the planet. This was an argument that could draw on notions of karma and divine retribution and the moral frame of Fairness and Cheating that is related to reciprocity. If the coronavirus was a form of

Citizens of Wuhan can finally hear birds chirping after years, Venice's water canals are clear and full of fish, and you can even see the Tatra mountains from Kraków because the smog has lifted.

This isn't an apocalypse. It's an awakening.

5:28 PM · Mar 17, 2020 · Twitter for iPhone

58.8K Retweets   **302.8K** Likes

Wow... Earth is recovering

- Air pollution is slowing down
- Water pollution is clearing up
- Natural wildlife returning home

Coronavirus is Earth's vaccine

We're the virus

8:25 AM · Mar 17, 2020 · Twitter for iPhone

70.9K Retweets   **290.9K** Likes

We. Are. The. Problem.

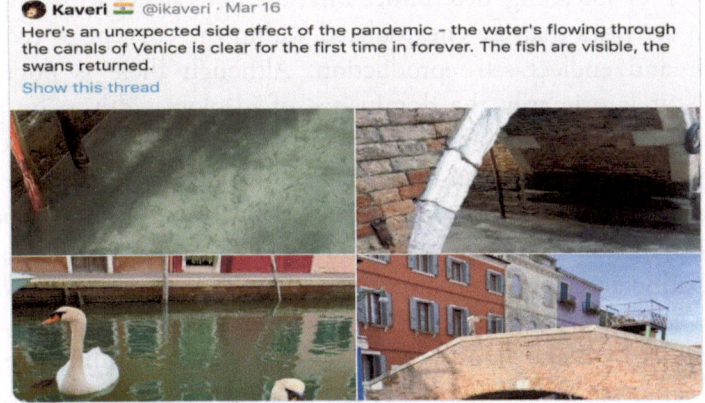

Kaveri 🇮🇳 @ikaveri · Mar 16
Here's an unexpected side effect of the pandemic – the water's flowing through the canals of Venice is clear for the first time in forever. The fish are visible, the swans returned.
Show this thread

1:41 AM · Mar 17, 2020 · Twitter for Android

409.2K Retweets   **1.4M** Likes

Fig. 4.2   Sample of "#We are the virus" Tweets

punishment in a time when God was no longer universally acknowledged as the agent of justice, the allegorical meaning was that nature had adopted this role. However, celebrating the strength of nature as a force for good that would restore the moral order assumed that the virus would *stop at man* and not go on to destroy other species. It assumed a moral order that exists *outside* of the human brain, whereas anyone who has watched nature in the raw, even a cat toying with an injured bird or mouse, knows that there is no room for fairness and the allegorical meaning of moral frames is essentially and definitively human. The law of nature is the law of survival. It was the desire to challenge the ecofascist ideologies behind such posts that led to the mutation of the 'We are the virus' meme by parody and satire. Blending analysis shows the conceptual basis underlying the multiplicity of arguments that could be drawn from the meme and in Fig. 4.3 I show how such a blending analysis might work:

My analysis of the metaphor places the virus in input space 1 as it is the main topic: the virus is now a way of commenting allegorically on humanity in input space 2. However, it is not every aspect of humanity that is commented on in the blend, but the damaging effect that humanity has on the environment. So various aspects of the generic space, such as the potential for spreading, determines what the virus shares with a range of human activities that are encapsulated within the concept of economic growth and endless self-reproduction. Although there is population growth, it is primarily the dominance of ideologies driven by profit-making that places economic growth as the exclusive determinant of success rather than, say, human well-being and happiness. Feeding the blend from the generic space is the knowledge that species exist in a competitive relationship with each other (unless mitigated by counter tendencies such as empathy) and only those species that show the attributes that warrant species survival are selected for genetic transmission. The virus treats the body as its food and flourishes as long as it has an ongoing supply of hosts—allowing the 'R' number to grow.[39] So, in the generic space, there is the notion of struggle, and the outcome of struggle selects those tendencies within the two inputs that comply with the survival of the fittest. The meme clearly does not profile human wellbeing as it argues for the need to eliminate humanity based on the survival of the fittest. The struggle of the virus causes the destruction of humanity and the survival of the planet.

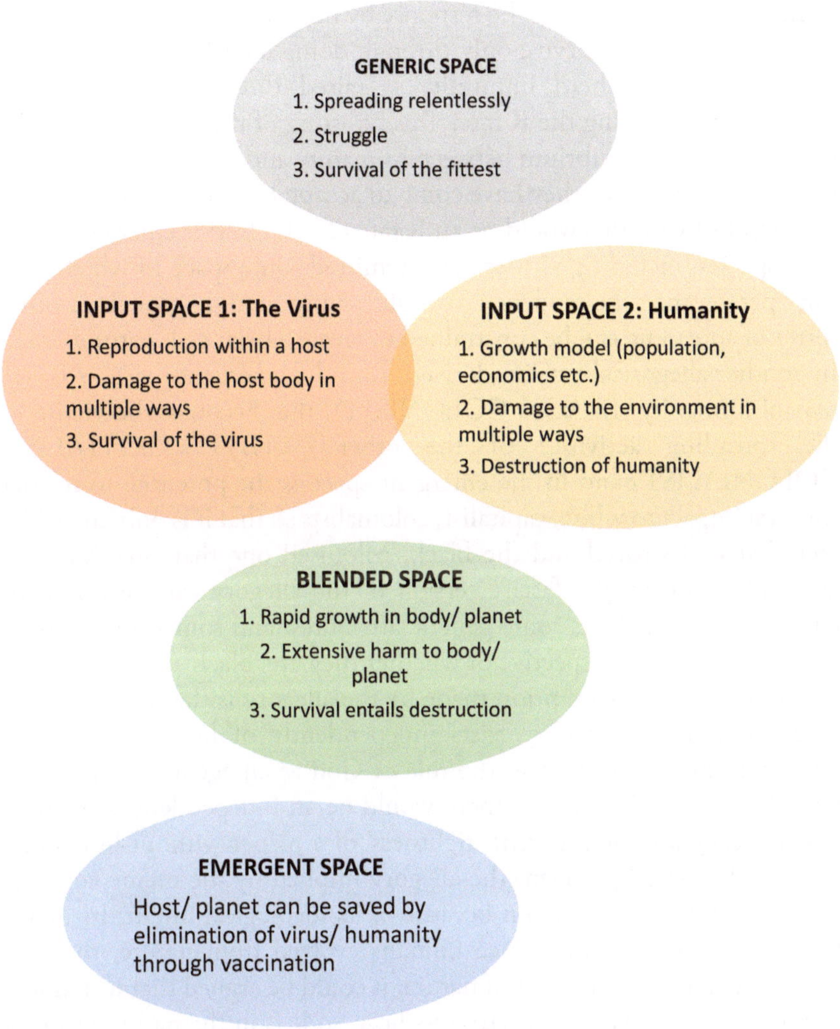

GENERIC SPACE

1. Spreading relentlessly
2. Struggle
3. Survival of the fittest

INPUT SPACE 1: The Virus

1. Reproduction within a host
2. Damage to the host body in multiple ways
3. Survival of the virus

INPUT SPACE 2: Humanity

1. Growth model (population, economics etc.)
2. Damage to the environment in multiple ways
3. Destruction of humanity

BLENDED SPACE

1. Rapid growth in body/ planet
2. Extensive harm to body/ planet
3. Survival entails destruction

EMERGENT SPACE

Host/ planet can be saved by elimination of virus/ humanity through vaccination

Fig. 4.3   Blending analysis of "We are the virus" meme

The survival of the fittest concept is the defining feature of eco-fascist ideology, because it views the virus as a form of nature that has been created to ensure its own survival by elimination of its primary challenger-mankind. As I have suggested, it is poorly conceived because if its food supply (i.e. humanity) dies out, then the virus goes with it.

In the emergent space is the response by humanity to the virus and the idea of how we can survive only through doing a deal with mankind in which humanity's herd immunity is raised through vaccination in exchange for lowering the R rate. This boosting of the antibodies creates some sort of an equilibrium between humanity and the virus so that they can both survive once they have come to acceptable terms (from humanity's point of view this would be an R rate of < 1). In this emergent space if all species, including viruses, are permitted some space in which they can operate, then the tendency to endless reproduction, growth or other forms of spreading can be constrained to create a balanced, natural order. In another allegorical version derived from the emergent space, it is one part of humanity (BLACK, COLONISED) that becomes the victim of the spreading activities of the other (WHITE, CAPITALIST, COLONIALIST) and in the emergent space is the potential to restrict the viral impact to white, capitalist, colonialists so that it is only the white race that is destroyed and the black, colonised one that survives. This alternative but equally fascist version of the allegory can be traced to eugenics that privileges some genetic attributes, and sometimes ethnicities, over others—irrespective of whether they are 'black' or 'white'.

A questionable assumption made by the allegory is that there is some form of moral order that exists independently of human cognition. Although the meme replaces the role of God as an agent of retribution with Nature, it still assumes there would be an independent consciousness to recognise the inherent 'rightness' of a planet without humanity. As it is ideologically driven, the allegory implied by the meme conceals many aspects of the situation because of its ideological intent. Its major blindness is the fact that since humans evolved from nature, they are necessarily and logically part of nature: it could be argued that just as it is in the nature of a virus to destroy its host, so it is in the nature of mankind to destroy its environment. This is a contested ideology because there is another version of man's relationship with nature in which it is through consciousness and scientific understanding of the impact of human behaviours on the environment, that humanity **can change its behaviours to create environmental balance and ensure survival**. In this allegory the emergent space would include vaccinations to build up human antibodies and the realisation that future viruses will continue to emerge unless the causes of zoonotic transmission are addressed- for example, by creating separation of species' habitats and ending deforestation. Viruses tend to stay within their hosts when their hosts are separate and only then can some sort of equilibrium exist between virus and host.

The way that the meme could be challenged was, typically, in the morality of social media, by parody: increasingly images depicting situations that were attributed to the restoration of a natural order in the original versions of the meme were replaced with a range of absurd images that parodied the idea of nature restoring itself. These included the return of dinosaurs, the return of giants, the return of Vikings in ships, the return of tigers to middle class lawns; the return of cows to the sea (with a photograph of a cow standing in the sea). Often there were digital mock-ups showing the return of the Lochness monster to Scotland or the return of daleks to British streets. Quite often the digital image might include a plastic animal toy of some sort, or even a large dildo, that was shown floating in water (one of the original memes was of dolphins returning to the bay of Venice). A meme depicted an inflatable crocodile in a swimming pool with a small 'real' crocodile on its back, another very popular one depicted lime green e-scooters dumped in the river. While most depicted animals, not all did, as one showed the return of supplies of toilet paper to the supermarket shelves and another the return of a stack of toilet bowls to a lawn. The rhetorical purpose of these parodies was to reframe the eco-fascist tendencies implicit within the meme. The 'We are the virus' meme advocated a laissez-faire attitude towards the virus: if it were doing a good thing by eliminating mankind then this was an endorsement of policies encouraged by leaders of nations such as Brazil and the US under Trump where mask wearing was discouraged and handshaking and proximity were seen as manifesting a human need to connect. Satirical versions of the meme inevitably undermined the illocutionary force of the original by framing it as simplistic and containing invalid, potentially fascist, arguments and therefore created a new allegorical meaning.

There has long been an eco-fascist tendency in certain areas of the environmental movement. One of the consequences of not addressing infection rates was that the virus spread much more rapidly amongst poorer people; in the western democracies these were associated with conditions such as obesity, and low health awareness, since good quality diet is viewed as less affordable than the fat-heavy diets promoted by capitalist advertising. Affordable housing was typically small and multi-generational and ethnicities associated with lower incomes and cultural preferences for extended family households within these small houses were more prone to infection. In international contexts it was the wealthier nations that could develop vaccinations and ensure their populations had first choice of them when they came on the market. So, eugenics came into the ideology of the 'We are the virus' thinking, in so far as it encouraged a laissez-faire attitude towards infection control measures allowing the poor to die out. Satirical tweets that commented indirectly on the implications of accepting the meme showed them to be absurd and lacking credibility. Nonetheless, there is no doubt that the meme must have encouraged a degree of fatalism and non-action to control the spread of the disease. But as Kenan Malek points out for *The Observer*:

> Humans are sinners not because we have disobeyed God but because we have violated nature, our teacher, in whose wisdom we must discover the moral rules by which we ought to live....The romanticisation of the "natural" is, Levinovitz notes, rooted in privilege. Only those who enjoy a life-style sufficiently protected from the ravages of nature have the licence to romanticise it. In countries with robust health systems, people have the dispensation to opt for natural childbirth, or alternative medicines, or reject vaccines. In much of the world in which "natural" childbirth is an imposition on women, not a choice, both maternal and infant mortality rates are staggeringly high. It is poverty that condemns so many in the global south to rely on traditional medicine or to live without vaccines.[40]

One reason that the meme spread so widely was because it appealed to multiple audiences according to different moral frames: for those concerned with Fairness, and more specifically, Cheating it was to fight a postcolonial battle against white supremacy to restore the moral order. For western environmentalists it was a call to arms against the harm that mankind had inflicted on the planet based on an appeal to the Sanctity of Nature and the Degradation of mankind, and for those with religious or spiritual viewpoints it was the moral frame of disgust at what man had done to the planet. In India and Sri Lanka this took on a particular cultural resonance as it was the harm done to elephants, accorded a sacred status in Hinduism, that was the prime motivation for the meme. Consider the following:

Heart shattered!! Pregnant #elephant Stuffed with #Crakers in #Kerala, She Died Standing In #River.[41] (2843 retweets, 4977 likes)

The tweet evoked extensive response:

Truly heart-wrenching! Humanity has died. No wonder we are being attacked by virus, locusts, earthquakes, thunderstorms. This is nature's way of saying #EnoughIsEnough. The world should come to an end already.

For your information don't mix religion and politics in everything, Just because it is malapuram, the people aren't inhumane. There will be some a**holes in every community.

There must be death penalty for those bastards it is the last limit of credulity

Who else is the perpetrators, Muslims, why no names are not coming out. Because it's secular crime?

Every year we offer payers to Ganesha. This year we killed a pregnant elephant…now am thinking that what lord Ganesha is thinking about this …

Human become so callous that he don't even care for innocent animal, and yet he expect nature to treat humanity in a better way Shame on humanity WeAReTheVirus.[42]

Intuitions based on the moral frames of Betrayal, Fairness and Cheating, and Sanctity and Degradation are all evident. The following account was offered by the BBC:

Wildlife officials in India are investigating the death of a pregnant elephant after it ate a pineapple containing firecrackers.
    The incident in Kerala caused outrage after a forest official posted about the death on social media. It's unclear if it was an accident, who planted the explosives or why. The animal spent days in pain before dying. Vets tried but failed to save her. India has some 27,000 wild elephants and another 2,500 in captivity.

Environment Minister Prakash Javadekar said the government had taken a "serious note of the killing". Kerala's chief minister says the investigation is focused on "three suspects", reports BBC Hindi's Imran Qureshi.

"Two suspects are being interrogated right now. We have not yet made any formal arrests," an official told the BBC.

Earlier the state forestry department had said there was no "conclusive evidence" to link the death to firecrackers, but most experts think the elephant ate what is called a "pig cracker", intended to scare wild boars away from crops.[43]

Apparently, this tragic event occurred when an elephant that was looking for food approached human habitats. A moral interpretation other than the one made on social media is that this was an accident caused inadvertently by a moral obligation of farmers to protect food sources threatened by animal intruders. However, it was not this moral frame that evoked emotions on social media, it was rather the display of feelings of disgust created by the idea of an elephant dying from an apparently wanton act of human cruelty. The cultural context of memes therefore strongly influences which *moral* frame will be evoked.

Unlike the 'zombie' meme where humanity could unite around opposing a common enemy, 'We are the virus' tweets created feelings of communal passion that was based on *reinforcing* 'Us' and "Them" relationships. This was evident with the tweeter who asked whether it was Muslims who had committed this moral offence. Nevertheless, what was going on here, in spite of the sectarian bias in some posts, was the creation of shared sentiment around the common moral emotion of Disgust. Overall, the 'We Are the virus' meme allowed expression of strong feelings that had been building up throughout the pandemic, yet it was not easy to vent them against a virus, however, a sense of disgust at mankind provided a safety valve for moral emotions that had become exclusively focused on the moral frame of Care and Harm. Restriction to a single moral emotion prevents the full expression of moral intuitions, especially among those not directly involved with social caring. There was a yearning for a more diverse range of moral sentiments and their corresponding allegories that contributed to a sense of identification with a group defined by religion, ethnicity, political orientation—or whatever else formed the mutual bond of connection with others. Social media provided the medium for this therapeutic role by communicating a wider range of moral emotions.

Notes

1. The Urban Dictionary defines 'doomscrolling' as "When you keep scrolling through all of your social media feeds, looking for the most recent upsetting news about the latest catastrophe."
2. https://twitter.com/JarettSays/status/1239714168065802241. Accessed 29 March 2021.
3. https://twitter.com/Davidlaz/status/1235671933699510272. Accessed 29 March 2021.
4. https://twitter.com/man_integrated. Accessed 29 March 2021.
5. https://twitter.com/comicsexplained. Accessed 29 March 2021.
6. https://twitter.com/unclerayscrazy. Accessed 29 March 2021.
7. *Express Online*, 18 January 2021.
8. https://www.english-corpora.org/corona/. Accessed 29 March 2021.
9. The Coronavirus Corpus is designed to be the definitive record of the social, cultural, and economic impact of the coronavirus (COVID-19) in 2020 and beyond. The corpus shows what people were saying in online newspapers and magazines in 20 different English-speaking countries. It was first released in May 2020 and was about 1045 million words in size on 6 June 2021.
10. Accessed 21 May 2021.
11. *The Independent*, 22 July 2020.
12. *Express Online*, 17 April 2020.
13. Accessed 21 May 2021.
14. *The Guardian (London)*, 12 October 2020.
15. *The Independent*, 29 April 2020.
16. Ho, J. & Chiang, E. (2021) 'Those lunatic zombies': The discursive framing of Wuhan lockdown escapees in digital space. In Musolff A., Breeze R., Vilar-Lluch S. & Kondon K. (eds.) *Pandemic and Crisis Discourse*. London: Bloomsbury. pp. 484–508.
17. Khan, A. (2021) Identity as Crime: How Indian mainstream media's coverage demonised Muslims as Coronavirus spreaders. In Musolff A., Breeze R., Vilar-Lluch S. & Kondon K. (eds.) *Pandemic and Crisis Discourse*. London: Bloomsbury. (pp. 514–538).

18. *Express Online*, 1 December 2020.
19. *The Guardian (London)*, 20 April 2020.
20. *telegraph.co.uk*, 7 August 2020.
21. *The Daily Telegraph (London)*, 7 March 2020.
22. *The Guardian (London)*, 14 November 2002.
23. *The Business*, 6 October 2002.
24. *The Daily Telegraph (London)*, September 2020.
25. *The Times (London)*, 20 November 2020.
26. *The Sunday Times (London)*, 5 April 52020.
27. *The Guardian (London)*, 24 September 2020.
28. *The Sunday Telegraph (London)*, 27 December 2020.
29. *telegraph.co.uk*, 5 October 2020.
30. *MailOnline*, 29 August 2020.
31. *The Times (London)*, 2 January 2021.
32. For a fuller account of blending theory please see Fauconnier, G. & Turner, M. (2002) *The Way we Think: conceptual blending and the mind's hidden complexities*. New York: Basic Books. And Charteris-Black, J. (2018) *Analysing Political Speeches: Rhetoric, Discourse and Metaphor*. Basingstoke & New York: Palgrave Macmillan. 2nd edition, pp. 231–241.
33. https://nurse.org/articles/nurses-viral-tiktok-social-media-covid19-videos/. Accessed 29 March 2021.
34. *Express Online*, 1 December 2020.
35. https://www.express.co.uk/news/science/721328/Zombie-outbreak-evolution-parasite. Accessed 29 March 2021.
36. https://www.bbc.co.uk/news/uk-england-bristol-51663632. Accessed 29 March 2021.
37. *The Guardian (London)*, 18 June 2020.
38. *The Observer (London)*, 10 May 2020.
39. The 'R' number is the number of people that an infected person will go to infect. For example, an R value between 1.2 and 1.4 means that, on average, every 10 people infected will infect between 12 and 14 other people.
40. *The Observer (London)*, 10 May 2020.
41. *Twitter*, 3 June 2020.
42. All posted on Twitter, 3 June 2020.
43. https://www.bbc.co.uk/news/world-asia-india-5291860. Accessed 29 March 2021.

5

Epidemiology: Science, and Metaphor

Introduction

In this chapter I explore a range of metaphors that were commonly used in public communication during the pandemic; these were frequently initiated in political communication and then reverberated around the press media to the extent that many became cliches. Such metaphor-based expressions include 'following the science', 'herd immunity', 'flattening the curve', 'spikes' and 'circuit breaker'. The government did not physically follow science, but rather it claimed to be heeding the advice of scientists, so there is a metonym here along the lines of PRODUCT (i.e. science) FOR PRODUCER (i.e. scientists). Many were metaphors that intended to make the science of epidemiology intelligible enough to encourage compliance with government guidelines although they were not always successful in doing this. In a survey conducted in January 2021, of the 2302 respondents, 90% had heard of 'herd immunity' but only 51% could confidently explain it (28% could explain it but not confidently).[1] The findings were similar for 'flatten the curve' and 'circuit breaker'. Overall, the percentages of people who could explain these metaphor-based terms were higher than for many literal Covid-19 terms

J. Charteris-Black, *Metaphors of Coronavirus*,
https://doi.org/10.1007/978-3-030-85106-4_5

that were included in the survey; for example, 49% had heard of 'epidemiologist' but could not explain it and only 44% could explain a 'PCR test'. I trace the origin of some metaphor-based scientific terms, provide an explanation of the rise and fall of their use during the Covid-19 pandemic and evaluate their rhetorical effectiveness in terms of moral framing, especially as regards Honesty and Dishonesty, which is a moral foundation that is not included in the social intuitionist model because of its exclusive reliance on the 'elephant' of intuition. I investigate both the *apparent* purpose of metaphor-based terms in making scientific concepts more accessible to the public and, more covertly, their less honest purpose of ameliorating the *blame* that was likely to be levelled at politicians.

'Following the Science' and 'Led by Science'

Of particular interest is a metaphor in which agency is attributed to 'Science', as noted by *The Times* (15th April 2020): "But how are politicians, especially those in power in these fraught times, going to respond? They keep telling us that their approach to this coronavirus crisis is always guided by what the science tells them". As an abstract entity 'Science' cannot 'tell' anyone anything, it is the scientists (and their communication advisers) who do the telling. Scientific opinion is typically divided and varied but such variations and divisions are obscured by metaphors that personify such as when 'The science tells us', or policies are claimed to be 'Science-led'. There was also something fundamentally ironic about appeals to 'the Science', since early on in the pandemic Boris Johnson's desire to shake hands with people was a behaviour that did not adhere to epidemiological advice and may have contributed to him getting coronavirus.[2] There may be good political and psychological reasons for shaking hands with strangers but they are not scientific ones. In this section I explore the ideological basis of tropes that attribute truth and authority to science and, specifically, epidemiology.

From the start of the pandemic the government based the legitimacy of its policies—especially those that placed constraints on personal freedom—by appealing to 'the science' as the basis for its decision making. In reality scientific opinion is rarely unanimous and there are different perspectives based on the methodologies or objectives of the research, but by paying homage to 'the science' government excluded any notion of debate *within* science; this oversimplification risked being dishonest. There are many different sciences—bioscience, epidemiology, behavioral and social psychology, sociology, statistics etc.—that could, and sometimes did, influence decisions and each of these could pull in different directions because of their epistemological differences. 'The science' is really a metonym for 'what scientists believe', based on PRODUCT FOR PRODUCER. However, to draw attention to such variation risked confusion and potentially non-compliance with government guidance. Although many could have understood the need for more nuanced messages, in the government's view, the overriding importance of the outcome would be undermined by lack of clarity. As a result, science was always referred to as 'the science'—with the definite article signaling unanimity of scientific opinion. Metaphors such as "following the science", which was used in 1065 press articles in the year after 1st February 2020, and "led by the science" (179 articles), profiled the agency of 'Science' rather than of politicians. A closely related metaphor 'driven by the science' (68 press articles) was employed as a variation that heightened the authority given to science and the constraints placed on politicians, a similar intention motivated 'governed by the science'. Table 5.1 shows the number of press stories in each month when the most common of these expressions occurred during the period 1st March 2020–28th February 2021:

I have treated the frequency of the press stories containing these expressions as an indication of their relative importance over time. The table shows that 'follow' or 'following the science' was the most preferred phrase followed by 'led by the science', although this expression had faded away by the autumn. It was used right from the start of the

Table 5.1 Metaphors appealing to 'science' in the British Press (2020–2021)

	Feb	March	April	May	June	July	Aug	Sept	Oct	Nov	Dec	Jan	Feb
Follow(ing) the science	2	66	112	179	93	65	47	99	144	68	63	77	45
Led by the science	0	17	58	37	0	1	11	11	4	9	6	4	2
Driven by the science	0	5	16	29	0	1	0	0	3	3	0	7	1

pandemic and before the announcement of Lockdown on 23rd March 2020:

> Speaking about the outbreak after being accused of acting to slowly, Prime Minister Boris Johnson said: "There's no question that this is going to become a significant, a much more significant outbreak than it currently is—that's obvious to everyone. But it is vital that we take the steps that we think are necessary at the right time and *we follow the science*."[3]

Sometimes the expression was used to contrast with other leaders who did not 'follow the science':

> Speaking before Mr. Trump's speech last night, Mr Johnson said: 'There's obviously people under a lot of pressure—politicians government around the world under a lot of pressure to be seen to act. So they may do things that are not necessarily *dictated by the science*. Boris Johnson swipes at leaders who *don't 'follow science'* on coronavirus.[4]

In his speeches Johnson tended to avoid 'follow the science' preferring to heighten further the agency of 'science':

> Throughout this period of the next two months we will be driven not by mere hope or economic necessity. We are going *to be driven by the science,* the data and public health.[5]

Here the use of the passive form 'to be driven' completely removes agency from the Prime Minister and hands it over to his Chief Scientific and Medical Officers: it enhances the power of the agonists. This triumvirate always worked well in distributing the blame for policies that often failed to stop the pandemic. The expressions 'follow' and 'led by' 'science' reached their peak in the early stages of responding to the first wave of the pandemic in April and May 2020. 'Following the science' was then revived during the second wave of the pandemic in September and October 2020 when further measures were introduced. Satirists sometimes passed comment on the endless reiteration of 'follow the science'— a cartoon by Matt was posted on Twitter showing a witch stirring a cauldron while casting a spell; the speech bubble reads: 'eye of newt, spleen of rat, leg of toad. Look I'm just following the science'. At times, the formulaic language of the trio of public officials did indeed sound like the incantation of three witches.

The expression 'following the science' was rarely used prior to the pandemic; the first instance in the British Press was in a quotation from Professor Robert Schoch of Boston University in 1995:

> I'm not saying that the Sphinx was built by Atlanteans or people from Mars, or extra-terrestrials. I'm just *following the science* where *it leads me*, and *it leads me* to conclude that the Sphinx was built much earlier than previously thought.[6]

It was used a little by politicians in relation to the foot and mouth outbreak in 2007:

> Mr Benn said: "People are at the site working very, very hard to find out. We are not dealing with certainty here but we have got the best people we can find who are doing the work and we will continue to *follow the science* at every stage."[7]

However, its use prior to 2010 was relatively infrequent. The instance of 9th March above is probably the first time that Johnson ever used the expression; in a book that I wrote about the metaphors of Brexit, I compiled press articles and speeches by Boris Johnson (120,000 words in total) and he did not once refer to 'the science'; he mentioned 'science' (no 'the') a very few times such as in the context of the contribution of bioscience to the economy. Had closer attention been paid to 'the science' it is possible that he, along with a number of other government ministers, would not have themselves contracted coronavirus and it was only *after* this experience that more than purely rhetorical acknowledgement was given to the advice of scientists regarding personal comportment. Truth and honesty contribute to survival and are therefore foundational to morality.

Some commentators challenged the claim that the government was indeed "following the science" as claimed:

> Richard Horton, chief editor of The Lancet, criticised the government's response, saying: "The UK government—Matt Hancock and Boris

Johnson—claim they are *following the science*. But that is not true. The evidence is clear. We need urgent implementation of social-distancing and closure policies. The government *is playing roulette* with the public. This is a major error."[8]

Here the speaker uses a different metaphor frame—gambling—to query the rhetorical claim to be 'following the science'. These criticisms grew extensively with the constant repetition of the phrase:

Experts have voiced growing frustration over the UK government's claim that it is "*following the science*", saying the refrain is being used to abdicate responsibility for political decisions. They also raised concerns that the views of public health experts were being overlooked, with disproportionate weight given to the views of modellers.

"As a scientist, I hope I never again hear the phrase 'based on the best science and evidence' spoken by a politician," Prof Devi Sridhar, chair of global public health at the University of Edinburgh, told the Guardian. "This phrase has become basically meaningless and used to explain anything and everything." government has repeatedly said it is being "*led by the science*" on decisions ranging from banning mass gatherings to closing schools, the use of face masks and, most recently, the prospects of lifting the lockdown. However, Sridhar and others argued that scientific views on these topics could be wide-ranging and dependent on a scientist's field of expertise.

The article goes on to argue that policy was based too much on binary choice of either eradicating the virus or allowing it to become endemic. Other experts noted that it was a very limited range of 'science' that was being followed, Prof Mark Woolhouse is reported as saying:

"What we're not talking about in the same formal, quantitative way are the economic costs, the social costs, the psychological costs of being under lockdown," he said. "I understand that the government is being advised by economists, psychiatrists and others, but we're not seeing what *that science is telling them*. I find that very puzzling. ... With any disease there is a trade-off. Public health is largely about that trade-off. What's happening here is that both sides of the equation are so enormous and so damaging that the routine public health challenge of balancing costs and benefits is thrown into incredibly stark relief. Yet that balance has to be found."[9]

Here an epidemiologist is suggesting that political decisions were over-dependent on epidemiology, rather than on economics or psychiatry. A correspondent to *The Independent* was equally critical:

The number of deaths has risen above 30,000 yet this government refuses to take responsibility nor offer an apology for its abject failures. They constantly claim they are "*following the science*" So, the science says forget the elderly in care homes and BAME cultures, does it? The science says deliberately deprive the NHS of funding and staff for 10 years then encourage us to clap for the staff?[10]

Even *MailOnline* joined in the chorus of criticism:

Ministers should stop claiming they are '*following the science*' and stop passing the buck in the battle against coronavirus, a leading scientist has demanded. Sir Adrian Smith, 73, a statistician and the incoming president of the Royal Society, said politicians are justifying their measures by saying they are *following expert advice* to appear decisive.[11]

As the second wave set in and keen not to miss out on the chorus of criticism, *The Express* followed suit:

But Boris was allowed to wriggle off the hook claiming he was *following the science*. A classic non-answer. Indeed "*following the science*" has predictably become every politician's go to when they have no real answer or indeed can weaponise the phrase to score political points.[12]

Eventually the attempt to avoid blame that appeared implicit in the phrase was exposed:

At last, the "*following the science*" myth is being punctured. Until now, the scientists and the politicians have broadly agreed on both "how" and "when" the rules should be relaxed. But a difference has clearly emerged over the "when." Some Sage members point out that today's change is a political decision.[13]

The government's scientific advisory committee known as SAGE were by this time frustrated by being held responsible for all decisions made by government and this is one reason that reference to 'The Science' was rapidly replaced by the slogan that policy would now be governed by 'Data not dates'; this was not used at all prior to February 2021; it was first quoted as follows:

> SAGE's Professor Stephen Reicher said timings "should be driven by *data not dates*."[14]

> Steve Chalke, chief executive of the Oasis academies trust … said he believed it was "impossible" to open all schools fully and urged a phased return with exam years brought back first. "We should be driven by scientific *data not dates*," he said.[15]

Enamoured of the alliteration, Boris Johnson soon picked up on the trope:

> The prime minister said: "The virus doesn't celebrate Easter. It's got to be about *data not dates*."[16]

And the slogan was soon taken as the basis for government policy:

> The case what Johnson allies call an approach based on "*data not dates*," is overwhelming.[17]

'Data not dates' did not occur at all in the British press in December 2020 or in January 2021, but by February 2021 the slogan had gone viral, appearing in 264 articles that month. Again, some of these were critical by pointing out that the claim that a policy based entirely on data was inconsistent with the so-called 'roadmap' out of lockdown that clearly did specify dates:

The prime minister's message that government policy around reopening would be guided by "*data not dates*" could be overshadowed by the use of dates in the roadmap, said Stephen Reicher ...

"*Data not dates* has turned into *dates not data*," said Reicher, who added that the choice of Midsummer Day for a possible return to normality was "incredibly powerful symbolic messaging". "Because, whatever you say, once you announce clear dates you create facts on the ground which alter the reality, and create a situation [where] it's very difficult to shift from those dates," he said.[18]

Evidently, government messaging needed to respond to the criticisms of 'follow the science' and this reflects in the reduction from 77 press articles in January 2021 to 45 articles in February; this was concomitant with the rise of 'data not dates'. At the end of his address to the nation in January 2021 announcing a further national Lockdown, Boris Johnson paid homage to science: "And, thanks to the miracle of science, not only is the end in sight and we know exactly how we will get there." Of course, miracles are one thing that science can't explain! However, it was concern with the *appearances* of Science, rather than its reality, that was his dominant concern. Appeals to 'the Science' had never characterised his rhetoric during the Brexit campaign when his various allegories had appealed to the moral frames of Liberty and Oppression, Fairness and Cheating, Care and Harm and Loyalty and Betrayal; together they had given voice to the emotional intuitions of Leave supporters, rather than dealing with the more reason-based arguments of the campaign. But now the rider of reason was regaining control over the elephant of intuition.[19]

Herd Immunity

On 13 March, The Chief Scientific Advisor, Sir Patrick Vallance told BBC Radio that one of "the key things we need to do" is to "build up some kind of herd immunity so more people are immune to this disease and we reduce the transmission".[20] 'Herd immunity' requires enough people to get infected for the whole group to develop immunity to the disease. Vallance said 60% of the UK's population would need to become infected for herd immunity to be achieved.[21] There was an outraged response when the possible scale of death that this entailed became evident and Matt Hancock denied that the government was pursuing a policy of 'herd immunity'. This outrage was because interpretations of the term assumed that 'herd immunity' implied a complacent attitude that relied on nature to take its course. Herd immunity is the indirect protection from an infectious disease that develops when a population becomes immune either because a previous infection has led to their immune systems developing antibodies **or through vaccination**. So when Hancock denied that the government was pursuing a policy of herd immunity it could imply that it was not seeking to vaccinate the population. All people who have antibodies through either natural means or vaccination serve as barriers to further infection of a population. If you have enough 'barriers' then the disease cannot spread effectively and over time the rate of infection will decline (the much quoted 'R' number) and the disease will fade away. So only a *proportion* of a population need to have developed antibodies for the *whole* population to have obtained a degree of immunity and a criticism of anti-vaxxers is that they are piggybacking on the antibodies developed through the vaccination of others.

The one-sided interpretation of 'herd immunity' as equivalent to a 'let it rip' policy made by those such as Matt Hancock, was in response to the interpretation of the term by libertarian supporters of the Great Barrington Declaration:

> As immunity builds in the population, the risk of infection to all—including the vulnerable—falls. We know that all populations will eventually reach *herd immunity*—i.e. the point at which the rate of new infections is stable—and that this can be assisted by (but is not dependent upon) a vaccine. Our goal should therefore be to minimize mortality and social harm until we reach *herd immunity*.

> The most compassionate approach that balances the risks and benefits of reaching *herd immunity*, is to allow those who are at minimal risk of death to live their lives normally to build up immunity to the virus through natural infection, while better protecting those who are at highest risk. We call this Focused Protection.

The Declaration again make no mention of vaccination and it is assumed that only two things are needed: development of natural immunity and protection of the vulnerable. Had its supporters placed greater emphasis on vaccination they may have won more support for their libertarian stance. Given the prominence given to the term, it is not surprising that 'herd immunity' shifted from being a scientific concept to an everyday expression. In the year prior to the pandemic it was only used five times in the British press, by contrast, during the year from 1st March 2020, it occurred 5137 times. Table 5.2 shows that it was frequently used in press articles throughout this period:

As previously mentioned, according to a survey of 2302 people 90% had heard the phrase 'herd immunity' but only just over 50% were confident that they could explain it, however 39% had heard it but could not explain it (either at all or confidently).[22] It was an important concept because it was closely related to views on the development of vaccination as a means of controlling the virus. 'Herd immunity' became a controversial expression because of the two different ways of obtaining herd immunity described above—either naturally through an earlier infection, or through vaccination. Some (a minority comprised mainly of libertarians) preferred immunity to arrive by *natural* means while others sought a *vaccine* as soon as possible. This was because allowing herd immunity to develop naturally would risk a death figure of as high as 500,000 and hence was politically unacceptable. I suggest that one of the reasons for the quite high number of people who were not confident that they could explain the meaning was because of a confusion between its literal and metaphoric senses. Although 'herd immunity' was first coined in epidemiology in 1923 the word 'herd' has a primary sense that refers to a large group of animals. It is quite commonly applied metaphorically to humans in expressions such as 'follow the herd' and when used in this way the term implies an exclusive focus on the collective rather than on the individual. This collective sense of equating humans with animals implies an absence of conscious autonomy, and agency, and so is pejorative.

Table 5.2 'Herd immunity' and 'cocoon' in the British Press (2020–2021)

	Feb	March	April	May	June	July	Aug	Sep	Oct	Nov	Dec	Jan	Feb
Herd immunity	1	722	776	501	248	253	206	346	528	315	376	466	375
Cocoon	8	130	118	134	75	33	31	29	61	22	32	73	27

The word 'vaccination' derives from the Latin vacca, 'cow', and much of the early resistance to vaccination derived from moral feelings about the threat to the sanctity of humans posed by injecting animal products into their bodies. As argued in chapter one, the imposition of the power of the state over personal autonomy motivated resistance to vaccination by arousing moral frames such as Authority and Subversion, Liberty and Oppression and Sanctity and Degradation. Although intended as a scientific concept, 'herd immunity' was interpreted by many as implying moral concepts and it is perhaps for this reason that they were not sure they could explain it; this may also be why use of the metaphor declined from May 2020. Even though it had returned by October with the onset of the second wave of infection, it did not rise to the same level as in the first wave. Conceptually 'herd immunity' is closely related to 'cocooning', because while immunity is being developed through natural immunity or vaccination, vulnerable people need to be protected; for this reason, the pattern of frequency of 'cocoon' in the number of press articles in which it occurs corresponds with that of 'herd immunity' (see Table 5.2). 'Cocoon' is discussed in more detail in Chap. 7.

Many commentators were highly critical of the 'herd immunity' metaphor, and this may have influenced the shift away from the term in the second wave; in an extended critical reflection on the language of the pandemic Robert Fisk makes highly satirical use of the metaphors HUMAN IS ANIMAL and ANIMAL IS HUMAN:

> …All of the above must be understood before we confront the on-again off-again policy of 'herd immunity' to which Boris Johnson and his medical chums were at one stage going to condemn their people. … I know that 'herd immunity' is an old medical term, but it is particularly pernicious now. Quite apart from the very word "herd"—which may indeed be the contemptuous expression which Johnson, Cummings and others use about UK citizens—the "immunity" which these cows/sheep/victims will enjoy can only be obtained by catching, suffering and in some cases dying of coronavirus.
>
> If there was a vaccine for Covid-19, the offered "immunity" might be more easily digestible even if members of the herd did not really understand its implications. But in the context of the coroner-doctor's early advice, the

immunity was clearly only to have been bought at a deadly price: with a cull of pensioners, the "elderly" or the old among the common herd. Or those who might be expendable enough—albeit not to "loved ones"—to expire "before their time".[23]

The moral frame of Care and Harm clearly overrides other considerations for Fisk. Animal metaphors were also noted by *The Guardian*:

For the government's hastily cobbled-together response to Covid-19, the metaphor "on the hoof" pleasingly echoes its original strategy, which it now denies was ever its strategy (it was), of aiming for "herd immunity" in the population. We might bristle at being portrayed as a nation of cows, but we are surely led by donkeys.[24]

Even if in fact the government was seeking to gain herd immunity in its technical sense by as early as mid-April 2020 it had partially abandoned this metaphor. The most common verbs preceding 'herd immunity' in a large corpus[25]–'achieve', 'create' and 'build'—are all positive words, and yet unconsciously, as noted by these commentators, the animal frame triggered a negative response and was more likely to encourage anti-vaccination sentiment. By this time, it was clear that the 'herd immunity' metaphor was to be avoided, and so Jonathan Van Tam, surreptitiously replaced 'herd' with 'community':

Professor Jonathan Van Tam, the deputy chief medical officer, has been the master of the metaphor when making the case for the vaccine. He uses another clever linguistic technique when he talks about how each person vaccinated contributes to *community immunity*. This is more persuasive and acceptable than suggesting individuals contribute to herd immunity, the inference of behaving like sheep isn't appealing.[26]

What is interesting in this regard is that someone who had a vital role in communicating the nation's medical policy recognizes just how important metaphor is in achieving its communication objectives of increasing the uptake of vaccination. His intentional and skilful employment of metaphor is noted by *the Guardian*:

One of the reasons Prof Jonathan Van-Tam is so popular as a scientific communicator is because he's a master of the metaphor. While Boris Johnson's metaphors tend to revolve around gauche world war two references which often seem inappropriate, Van-Tam's have been applauded. This morning the Today programme even broadcast a compilation. Radio 4's Today programme currently doing a mash-up of Jonathan Van-Tam's pandemic metaphors. In his Q&A on BBC Breakfast, Van-Tam explained how he acquired this habit. He said:

I began testing them [his metaphors] many years ago, and I hope he won't mind me saying—I don't suppose he is a lance corporal any more—but L/Cpl Andy Lennox, if he's listening, was one of the great people that used to ask me medical questions as we sat around tents in Snowdonia. And I practised the art there, I suppose, of turning medicine into stories, if I could. And with my family too—Mrs VT is very good at listening to all that stuff … Rachel Burden, the Radio 5 Live presenter, said she had never seen so many listeners submit questions for a guest—even when she had had the prime minister in the studio.[27]

It is significant that the reference to the tiredness of Boris Johnson's World War Two metaphors was something that my informants commented on in the survey (see Chap. 2) and this contrasted with a more diverse and varied use of metaphor by Van-Tam that led to the coining of a nickname 'Mr Metaphor' in the tabloid press:

Jonathan Van-Tam A much-needed injection of charisma into the government press conferences, JVT's straight talking was a welcome relief from the waffling men in suits next to him.
    Also known as Mr Metaphor, he's put his pandemic point across using analogies about trains, penalties, hosepipes, planes and yogurt.[28]

Van Tam's metaphors in relation to the vaccine are discussed further in Chap. 9. Further suspicion accrued to the herd immunity metaphor once some 'anti-vaxx' myths suggested that the vaccine contained animal products; of course, pork products were a particular concern for Muslim communities, and 'anti-vaxx' vloggers were quick to exploit these fears, as the Guardian noted:

The Guardian has been sent a number of other videos posted by different individuals, some standing outside vaccination centres, as they discuss unsubstantiated claims that the vaccine might contain pork, is not halal or that it could result in modification of DNA playing on religious concerns.[29]

In fact, it was the failure of the government to explain fully that herd immunity relied just as much (if not more) on vaccination than it did on natural immunity that gave the opportunity for 'anti-vaxxers' to equate 'herd immunity' with an anti-vaccine position:

At the conference, Del Bigtree, a prominent US anti vaxx activist, summarized a three-point strategy for undermining public faith: "It's dangerous. You don't need it. And herd immunity is your friend," he said, according to the report.[30]

Here the 'anti-vaxx' activist readily equates herd immunity with the non-interventionist, let it rip message of 'anti-vaxx', and clearly does not understand that 'herd immunity' relies as much on vaccine development as it does on natural immunity.

The government switched away from 'herd immunity' as a term in public communication, though not as a concept, after April 2020 because they realized that since 'herd' was associated with 'animals' when it was used to refer to humans it took on a negative semantic prosody.[31] For example, when looking in a large sample of language we find that a very common expression is 'herd mentality'—'mentality' is in fact the third most frequent word following 'herd' (after 'immunity' and 'cattle'), and always has a negative meaning:

It's mindless conformity, quite frankly, *herd mentality*, and I just could not tolerate it.

For Edmundson football is "potentially ennobling, potentially toxic" it can breed "brutality, thoughtlessness, dull conformity, love for the *herd mentality* and the herd".

Although 'herd immunity' is more common than 'herd mentality', they are the two most frequent non-literal collocations of 'herd' in English. Another negative metaphoric expression is 'herd behaviour' as in:

> The best weapon against mindless *herd behaviour* is the human mind. Don't just teach kids how to make Web sites; teach them how to think.[32]

The semantic prosody of 'herd' when used as a metaphor referring to human behaviour is negative, as it implies an absence of individual, 'human' thought and reliance on emotional responses alone. It is perhaps for this reason that the confusion of the 'herd immunity' with 'herd mentality' by Donald Trump was extensively reported in the British and the American press:

> Donald Trump claimed Tuesday during a televised town hall that "herd mentality" could make the coronavirus "disappear" with or without a vaccine. During a 90-minute town hall hosted by ABC News in the must win battleground of Pennsylvania, Trump defended his repeated assertion that the virus will eventually disappear even without a vaccine, citing what he called "herd mentality" an apparent reference to "herd immunity". "Herd mentality", also known as mob mentality, rather means people can be influenced by the "herd" to act in ways that are emotional.[33]

Perhaps, since much of his support relied on the 'herd mentality' of unreflective emotional connection among himself and his followers, the confusion is indicative of an unconscious conflation of the two terms in his mind. In a flurry of metaphors, the journalist in the following extract plays around with the negative sense of 'herd mentality' in a rhetorical argument that rejects the concept of 'herd immunity':

> But as a No 10 official explained for the umpteenth time: Our objective is not to secure herd immunity. Our objective is to *flatten the curve* of the virus's spread to ensure the NHS and other services retain the capacity to protect the most vulnerable patients. ... The danger we face as a nation is not that we will be killed by a misguided policy on *herd immunity*. What is imperilling us is *a herd mentality*. A *stampede* away from facts and truth towards biases and prejudices embedded by years of *Brexit trench-warfare*.

It means shaking off the *herd mentality* and learning about *herd immunity*—educating ourselves about the way this is transmitted.[34]

Here the journalist ridicules the 'herd immunity' metaphor by extending it with 'herd mentality' and 'stampede'. He also introduces 'flattening the curve', a metaphor that I will consider next.

'Flattening the Curve', 'Squashing the Sombrero' and 'Spikes'

It is perhaps because of the semantic problems with 'herd immunity' that while the government continued to pursue herd immunity through vaccination it decided to supplement terms originating in epidemiology with those drawn from statistics, especially ones that could be reinforced by visual metaphors from graphs. 'Flattening the curve', 'squashing the sombrero' and other colourful versions such as 'the hump of the dromedary' were all novel metaphors based on the shape of line graphs displaying data on Coronavirus. These were widely used to refer to the numbers of cases and fatalities on the y-scale and time on the x-scale; in the year from 1st March 2020 'flatten the curve' or 'flattening the curve' was used in 2063 press reports. The 'flatter' the curve meant the longer the period of time over which the same number of infections were incurred and so increased the likelihood of hospitals being able to cope with demand.

In the survey referred to above, 89% had heard 'flatten the curve' but only 48% were confident that they could explain it, with a higher proportion of males (53% as compared with 43% females). Awareness of the expression may be explained by exposure in the press as 'flattening the curve' or 'flatten the curve' occurred in 461 articles in March 2020 and had risen to 680 articles in April which indicates that its use was growing rapidly although it was not yet fully understood as a concept (see Table 5.3).

Initially this new metaphor appeared in speech marks:

In simple terms it aims to delay and "*flatten the curve*" of the epidemic if it hits Britain. It means taking measures which prevent the virus running

Table 5.3 Immunity-related metaphors in the British Press (2020–2021)

	Feb	March	April	May	June	July	Aug	Sept	Oct	Nov	Dec	Jan	Feb
Flatten(ing) the curve	1	461	680	244	88	92	42	80	79	33	45	14	13
Squash(ing) the sombrero	0	36	26	27	6	0	0	2	12	3	2	2	1
Spike in	1213	1020	1080	1213	1373	1975	1488	1465	964	656	768	540	486

through the population at speed and unhindered so the impact is spread over time and the NHS is not overwhelmed.[35]

Sometimes there was a definition:

Much of the impact will depend on how well the public health measures being put in place can "*flatten the curve*"—spreading out cases so that they do not all arrive at once and overwhelm hospitals.[36]

Or an explanation of the metaphor;

Lockdowns, self isolations and social distancing tactics have helped China "*flatten the curve*" referring to the shape of the line on graphs plotting the numbers of cases of the disease over time.[37]

The trope here is one in which abstract measurement by numbers becomes a legitimate 'scientific' trope through visual representation using the conventions of the line graph. It is suggested that this is because numeracy was not assumed by policy communicators and therefore required a more accessible visual representation. This also motivated another metaphor:

flatten the curve—or as Boris Johnson put it "*squash the sombrero*"— though, and even if the same number are infected far fewer die. Faced with fewer infections at the same time, the NHS has enough respirators and beds.[38]

"Squashing the sombrero" referred to the hat-shaped curve of the now famous flattening-the-curve graph. Boris Johnson introduced the metaphor of 'squash the sombrero' at his second press conference about the virus (12th March 2020) which used a representation of the 'flatten the curve' graph in the background to make it more intelligible and humorous:

> "We need to *flatten the curve, squash the sombrero*," he said, with the faintest hint of a smile. He tried to be upbeat in promising the country was making "huge strides" in getting enough ventilators, and allowed himself to hold out the prospect of eventual "remedies—even a vaccine".[39]

The two phrases were used interchangeably with the same meaning, although the replacement of 'curve' with 'sombrero' is a more innovative metaphor. In 'flatten the curve' is it only the verb 'flatten' that is a metaphor, as 'curve' literally refers to the shape of the line graph and follows the concept MORE IS UP, whereas the whole phrase 'squash the sombrero' is a metaphor. The drift from the literal towards metaphoric, from 'herd immunity', to 'flatten the curve', to 'squash the sombrero' indicates both the Prime Minister's own preference for metaphor, and the need to shift to a style of public communication that was believed to be more culturally accessible, although some may have found it patronising.

Always keen to combine humour with vigorous and innovative imagery, in September 2020 Boris Johnson introduced a new metaphor to describe the shapes made by graphs showing Coronavirus cases:

> Mr Johnson said: 'All this is to say that: Christmas we want to protect, and we want everyone to have a fantastic Christmas.
>
> 'But the only way to make sure the country is able to enjoy Christmas is to be tough now. So if we can *grip it* now, *stop the surge, arrest the spike, stop the second hump of the dromedary, flatten the second hump.*
>
> 'dromedary or camel? I can't remember if it is a dromedary or a camel that has two humps? Umm. Please check.
>
> 'Anyway *a double hump.* So that is what we need to do!'[40]

The flurry of metaphors in which the image of the camel riding alongside the lesser-known dromedary (also known as 'the one humped

Arabian camel'), is amusing and was in keeping with the jocular, optimistic tone preferred by Johnson. Unfortunately, his optimism was misplaced as he was later obliged by the arrival of new variants of the virus to impose a tight Lockdown 5 days before Christmas which disrupted most people's travel plans as well as ruining their Christmas. The metaphor has all the characteristics of embodiment that have marked out Johnson's style (see Charteris-Black 2019, chapter 6): the idea of 'gripping' the virus is a reification that makes it appear a concrete entity and the listing of paraphrases 'stop the surge etc.' is a reiteration that entertains by a display of mixed metaphors. Similarly, the interjection where he queries the meaning of 'dromedary' introduces the conversational style that he prefers to the more formal register imposed by the exigencies of the pandemic—particularly on the rather tedious Daily Coronavirus Briefings from Downing Street. BBC One broadcast these live as part of a *BBC News Special* programme from 16 March, doing so every day until the weekend briefings ceased towards the end of May, and finally stopped altogether on 23 June.[41]

'Spike' is another expression used extensively in statistics to refer to a rapid increase and also has metaphoric origins because its primary sense refers to a thin pointed piece of metal, wood or other rigid material. Its statistical sense has grown increasingly in recent years, as Table 5.4 shows, the word in general has become more frequent from 2010 onwards:

The corpus of American English (one billion words) also shows that 'spike in' has more than doubled in use between 2007 and 2019. Its use in the British press increased in 2014 in the reporting of various pandemics such as Middle Eastern Respiratory Syndrome and Ebola in Africa:

> *A spike in* the number of infections from a deadly virus that has now killed more than 100 people in Saudi Arabia is "concerning" but the risk to the UK remains low, health officials have said.[42]

Table 5.4 Frequency of 'spike in' in the British Press (2010–2020)

	2010	2011	2012	2013	2014	2015	2016	2017	2018	2019	2020
Spike in	644	1040	1786	2031	2364	2823	5644	3171	3686	3288	>10,000

But despite *a spike in* sales of surgical masks, and the hurried cancellation of thousands of holidays to Hong Kong and Thailand, the disease ended up killing only 775 people worldwide.[43]

Because of the familiarity of its abstract meaning of 'sudden increase' most linguists would consider this a case of polysemy when a particular word has more than one meaning. Here the senses are related because the shape of a sudden increase when represented on a graph resembles that of a spike. However, there are some interesting collocations of the word that indicate that it is nearly always followed by a negative entity of some sort. For example, in a general corpus one of the most common subjects is 'violence' as in:

One consequence of the new dominance of Mexican cartels is a *spike in violence*, especially along the 2000-mile US-Mexico border where rival cartels are warring not only against Mexican and US authorities.

The death of Egyptian soldiers caught in a battle between Israeli troops and Palestinian militants is testing the two nations landmark 1979 peace treaty, just as a sudden *spike in violence*. Saturday threatened to trigger a full-scale conflict between Israel and Gaza militants.

Other common collocations are 'oil prices' and 'idiosyncratic risk'. Apart from words directly related to Covid-19, another large corpus also shows negative entities tend to be described as 'spiking', these include 'worries', 'crime' and again 'violence'.[44] Do language users unconsciously prefer 'spike in' to the more literal 'increase' or partially more literal 'rise' because the word carries the negative semantic prosody of danger, threat and fear? Or it just that 'spike' is a somewhat 'edgy' word which increases its potential to grab attention around statistics that might otherwise appear tedious? The frequency of 'spike in' itself *spiked in* around July 2020, but from then on its use declined and, as it did so, broadened to a wider range of negatively evaluated phenomena as illustrated in the following from February 2020:

says stockpiling in the early weeks of the pandemic caused a subsequent *spike in* **food waste** from households.

At least 20 people were killed in three bombings on Saturday and Sunday, a *spike in* **violence** in a corner of the country that Turkey.

The Office for National Statistics (ONS) said there had been a statistically significant *spike in* **alcohol deaths** in the period after the first coronavirus lockdown was imposed.

The recent attacks represent the latest *spike in* **verbal and physical attacks** against Asian Americans since the coronavirus, which emerged in China, reached the United States.

So the 'spike in' metaphor that was widely employed in relation to Covid-19 in the context of 'cases', 'infections' 'deaths' semantically broadened to other negative social phenomena associated with pain and suffering. This was probably because 'spike in' itself primes the audience for negative senses as it is never used to refer to an increase in anything socially appealing.

The appearance of the language of science always had a key role for Johnson, especially as regards the tone of his expression. In a televised speech to the nation made on 22nd September 2020 he drew on another graph related metaphor:

We can see what is happening in France and Spain, and we know, alas, that this virus is no less fatal than it was in the spring, and that the vast majority of our people are no less susceptible, and *the iron laws of geometrical progression are shouting at us from the graphs* that we risk many more deaths, many more families losing loved ones before their time;

Following this rather elaborately mixed metaphor, he went on to issue his instructions:

So today I set out a package of tougher measures in England—early closing for pubs, bars; table service only; closing businesses that are not covid secure; expanding the use of face coverings, and new fines for those that fail to comply; and once again asking office workers to work from home if they can while enforcing the rule of six indoors and outdoors.[45]

The ratchetting up of measures of social control in his quest to contain the pandemic was prefaced by the somewhat confused metaphor: as with 'following the science' the images of "iron laws of geometry" and "shouting graphs" remove agency from himself as Prime Minister and imply that the responsibility for decisions about Coronavirus policy lies with the laws of the universe, as interpreted by his Chief Medical Officer and Chief Scientific Advisor.

Circuit Breaker

The expression 'circuit breaker' was used in 2652 British press articles during the one-year period after 1st March 2020. As with 'herd immunity' and 'flattening the curve', from very limited use in February 2020 it soon went *viral* as we can see from Table 5.5:

'Circuit breaker' featured in only two articles in February 2020, and one of these was literal and the other was in the context of a climate change debate, it had risen to 62 articles by March 2020, but none of these were with the metaphoric meaning it would acquire—a short Lockdown. At this time 'circuit breaker' had a metaphoric sense referring to the control of market trading:

> The S&P 500 fell by more than eight percent which kicked into gear what is known as *a circuit breaker*—a mechanism which acts like a kill switch to stop trading before prices can fall by too much.[46]

Yet less than a year later, 77% of a sample of over 2302 people indicated that they could explain it (48% confidently). Clearly people were learning the new language of the pandemic. A circuit breaker is a term used in electrical engineering to refer to an automatic safety mechanism whereby when there is as electrical overload there is a break in the circuit;

Table 5.5 'Circuit breaker' in the British Press (2020–2021)

	Feb	March	April	May	June	July	Aug	Sept	Oct	Nov	Dec	Jan	Feb
Circuit breaker	2	62	12	9	5	3	4	227	1517	369	194	163	130

this is usually by a fuse automatically flipping. When first used as a metaphor 'circuit breaker' was used in the context of market trading as in the above example; when panic effects of excessive market trading were causing excessive volatility, the authorities would force trading to stop. In relation to the Coronavirus pandemic, the metaphor was explained by *The Express Online*:

> But what exactly is a *circuit breaker*? A *circuit breaker* is an automatic switch which is installed in electrical circuits which flips and breaks the flow of electricity where there is a power surge or a short-circuit. In terms of a covid-lockdown, a *circuit breaker* would essentially see Britons cut almost all contact with anyone outside their household by shutting down non-essential businesses and banning social interactions.[47]

So how did a metaphor originating from electrical engineering become readily intelligible to over three quarters of the sample surveyed in such a short period of time? The metaphor originated in the United States during market volatility in 1987 and was first used in the British press in 1988:

> *Circuit-breaker* mechanisms, such as price limits and co-ordinated trading halts, should be implemented to protect the market system.[48]

Market trading has always been a hot bed for metaphor innovation with expressions such as 'dead cat bounce', and 'white knight'. It took quite a long time for the metaphor to broaden its range beyond financial trading, and the next domain that it was extended to was sport:

> In fairness, things have got a bit better recently and I think the decision by FIFA to give automatic qualification for the next World Cup to an Oceanic country was a *circuit-breaker* of a decision.[49]

> But Hamilton can help *circuit-breaker* Bernie lap up atmosphere *circuit-breaker* Bernie lap up atmosphere.[50]

The first use in the domain of politics that I have found was in 2009:

Peter Moore is believed by all sides to be alive. His freedom will probably require a *circuit breaker*: freedom for Qais al-Ghazali.[51]

The idea here is of a way of finding a non-financial resolution to a problem in the form of an exchange of a political prisoner. It was only gradually and after the period of financial austerity that the metaphor broadened to this wider sense of making a political breakthrough:

> The EU pushed the government and parliament into agreeing a second austerity package on June 29, in return for the promise of a new (EURO) 159 billion bail-out. That was supposed to be the *circuit breaker*...[52]

Here the idea of 'circuit' breaker seems to merge with that of 'deal breaker' and it may well be that the latter derived from the former. Nevertheless, since over 90% of the uses of 'circuit breaker' prior to 2020 were literal it can be considered a novel metaphor. A broader shift to metaphoric uses was not until 2015 when in relation to same sex marriage, Australians were informed that:

> The independent senator Nick Xenophon says a referendum here would be a "*circuit breaker*".[53]

In Australia the expression developed as a metaphor:

> Reading that scoutmaster Rod Corrie, the man who he said inappropriately touched him, had been jailed for abusing other children over a 30-year period, was the *circuit breaker* he needed to speak out and seek help.[54]

The use in Australia is probably because the dual interest in sports and finance created the opportunity for the expression to take on broader meanings such as the above. In Britain from around this time the metaphor also extended to politics:

> The purpose of the marathon press conference in the old days was a means of clearing static. Clearly Abbott is looking for a *circuit breaker*. Doing the press conference this morning is a billboard sized marker: we are in trouble, I know we are in trouble.[55]

In relation to Covid-19 policy the 'circuit breaker' metaphor was sometimes explained by analogy with the more familiar metaphor of 'fire-breaker':

A *circuit breaker* or "*fire-breaker*" lockdown will come into force at 6 pm on Friday in Wales. Pressure from scientists and other experts is growing on the Government to impose a short-term "*circuit-breaker*" lockdown in England as coronavirus cases continue to rise.[56]

Ms. Sturgeon said that "whether you call it a *circuit breaker* or a *fire breaker* ... that is the kind of thing that I think we're all thinking about just now."[57]

It is worth pausing for a moment to consider why 'circuit breaker' became preferred to 'fire breaker'. On reason may be that in the UK as forest fires are not particularly common, the concept of a circuit breaker is simply more familiar than 'fire breaker'; evidence for this is found in the fact that some newspapers found a need to define 'fire breaker':

A "*fire-break*" lockdown is the exact same thing as a "*circuit breaker*" lockdown. Put simply it's a "*short and sharp*" lockdown, similar to the national lockdown in March—but this time just for Wales.

Usually, a "fire breaker" is an obstacle that stops the spread of a fire, such as a large open space in a forest.

A "*fire breaker* lockdown" will theoretically act in a similar way and involves a set of measures which will be in place to stop the spread of Covid, save lives and prevent the NHS from being overwhelmed. Labour leader Keir Starmer explained a *circuit break* lockdown as "a temporary set of clear and effective restrictions to get the R rate down." [58]

Here the author finds it necessary to explain a 'fire breaker' but assumes that the reader knows what a 'circuit breaker' is. It is worth noting that in the survey 52% of males were confident that they could explain 'circuit breaker' whereas only 44% of women shared the same confidence.

Similarly, the understanding appears to have been higher in Northern Ireland (64%) and Scotland (56%), Wales (51%) than in England (46%). This was probably because it was used more by the regional assemblies in those parts of Britain, for example in October 2020 a 'circuit breaker' Lockdown was imposed in Northern Ireland whereas Boris Johnson rejected the calls for a similar one in England instead preferring to introduce a tier system.

'Circuit breaker' was first used as a metaphor in relation to Covid-19 in April 2020 when on reporting Singapore's response to the outbreak Antonia Syn wrote:

> Only last week a full lockdown was announced, working as a *'circuit breaker'* to slow the spread.[59]

The term 'circuit breaker' as a description of a political policy therefore developed in Singapore but was reported on in the British press:

> The plan is the first phase of lifting of Singapore's so-called *"circuit breaker"* restrictions to stem the spread of the coronavirus, which expire on 1 June.

I suggest that the 'circuit breaker' concept in political contexts has its origin in the discourse of the founding leader of Singapore Lee Kuan Yew who showed an affection for electricity-based metaphors as long ago as 1977:

> For us, the easier way is just to *plug it into the grid*. We stand other risks, of course, because *the grid is already there*, You tap Western science, Western technology, trade with the West. But when they have a depression, recession and unemployment, we get the rigor.[60]

This was not a one-off metaphor either, in 1985 he reiterated it on a number of occasions:

> Hong Kong and ASEAN have had from the free market economies of the West by *plugging into their trading and investments power grid*.[61]

The analogy between the flow of knowledge and the flow of money was a powerful one that corresponded well with the new emphasis on science and technology around which the Singaporean economy was being developed. In relation to Covid-19 the 'circuit breaker' metaphor originated in Singapore and both the metaphor and the concept were then borrowed into British political discourse in articulating a policy for pandemic control. This origin was acknowledged in some of the British press:

> The notion of a *circuit breaker*—or partial lockdown—can be traced to Singapore, where it saw schools and all but essential workplaces closed, as well as restrictions on restaurants and other public places.[62]

By mid-October the metaphor had become an established concept in political discourse and, as we have seen, was introduced as a policy by some of the regions:

> The idea of a *circuit breaker* was also backed by metro mayors in northern England provided it came with more financial support than is currently on the table. The mayors of Greater Manchester, the Sheffield city region and North of Tyne represent a combined 5.5 million people.
> Andy Burnham, mayor of Greater Manchester, said he would prefer a nationwide *circuit breaker* to tier 3 ("very high risk") measures because it "would be much more effective, come with proper financial support and allow the reset of test and trace".[63]

> Starmer had urged the government on Tuesday to "follow the science" and impose a *circuit breaker* of at least two weeks to stem the spread of Covid-19. Starmer's intervention followed the release of advice from the government's Sage committee, which warned ministers … that the country faced a "very large epidemic with catastrophic consequences" unless they took immediate action by imposing a two-week *circuit breaker*.[64]

Why is it that a relatively novel metaphor went through an accelerated spread, broadening out from its conventional use in financial trading, via sports, to refer to a specific policy response to a pandemic? 'Metaphors such as 'flatten the curve' and 'squash the sombrero', although colourful, were directed towards *describing* the spread of Covid-19 rather than addressing its *causes and the necessary actions*. Looking at the shape of line graphs showing increases in cases, deaths from Covid 19 etc. is an *after the event* descriptive approach whereas Covid policy needs to recommend *actions* taken *in anticipation of* a rise in the number of infections.

The 'circuit' breaker metaphor is action-oriented and encourages the listener to reflect on cause-effect relationships rather than simply describing the reality of increased infections. The electricity in this metaphor is the rise in infections, with the implied meaning that social interaction between people leads to an increase Covid-19 infection. The 'circuit breaker' response explains how it is necessary to react with an instant, brief Lockdown. Data doesn't change in graphs until several weeks *after* a virus-control policy, but electricity stops *immediately* the electrical circuit is broken. It also conveys other aspects of the domain of electricity that readily assist in understanding disease: electricity is known to be dangerous, and because it is dangerous it requires an automatic response. It does not mean that electricity will not flow again once the fuse switch is flicked back but it suggests something that is easy, fast, efficient and easy to reverse. It is also technical in nature, and it brings with it the authority of everyday knowledge of science—this is quite different from 'dromedaries' and 'sombreros' which tend to belittle the virus transmission by treating it as a topic for comic relief. It avoids evoking unhelpful emotions and reestablishes the rider of reason in control over the elephant of intuition.

Finally, since the term 'circuit breaker', is quite familiar though not especially frequent in the language, it seems commentators were not particularly aware of it being a metaphor; in articles published in the period March 2020–2021 that refer to both 'metaphor' and 'circuit breaker' none refer to 'circuit breaker' as a metaphor, instead discussing other metaphors such as 'fire-breaker'. Initially, there were speech marks put around the metaphor and it was prefaced by the adjectives 'short' and 'sharp'. This is the practice of selective quotation. This suggests that, like the metaphoric use of 'viral', the cognitive efficacy of the metaphor facilitated its uptake and spread. The phrase also alludes to the alliterative phrase 'short, sharp shock'. Common collocations following 'circuit breaker' were 'kicked in' and 'was triggered' that attribute agency to the 'circuit breaker'. When something 'kicks in' it means that we don't have any control over it, as when people talk of their 'instincts' or 'training' kicking in with the sense that these are *automatic responses* over which the have *no conscious control*. So, if a circuit breaker 'kicks in', it therefore reduces the identity of the person or group who has decided that a Lockdown of this type is necessary and avoids evoking unnecessary moral intuitions. The removal of human agency and the idea that the onset of a Lockdown was mechanical and automatic and was attractive to decision-makers as a means of avoiding blame for taking reason based decisions that, though unpopular to many and uncomfortable for all, derived from the rider of reason.

Notes

1. https://2sjjwunnql41ia7ki31qqub1-wpengine.netdna-ssl.com/wp-content/uploads/2021/01/MHP_Public-Poll-Covid-Terms_Tables_20-01-21.pdf. Accessed 24 June 2021.
2. "A newly-published document by the Independent Scientific Pandemic Influenza Group on Behaviours (SPI-B), a sub-group of the Sage advisory panel, reveals officials agreed to "advise against" hand shakes on 3 March. That was the same day the Prime Minister told a Downing Street press conference: "I was at a hospital the other night where I think a few there were actually coronavirus patients. "And I shook hands with everybody, you'll be pleased to know, and I continue to shake hands." https://www.politicshome.com/news/article/boris-johnson-boasted-of-shaking-hands-with-coronavirus-patients-on-same-day-officials-urged-ban-new-documents-show.
3. *Daily Star Online*, 9 March 2020.
4. *MailOnline*, 12 March 2020.
5. Prime Minister's statement, 10 May 2020.
6. *Daily Mail*, 5 April 1995.
7. *Guardian.com*, 6 August 2007.
8. *Daily Mirror*, 12 March 2020.
9. *The Guardian*, 23 April 2020.
10. *The Independent*, 8 May 2020.
11. *MailOnline*, 19 May 2020.
12. *Express Online*, 27 January 2021.

13. *The Independent*, 1 June 2020.
14. *The People*, 7 February 2021.
15. *The Sunday Times*, 14 February 2021.
16. *thetimes.co.uk*, 21 February 2021.
17. *The Independent*, 16 February 2021.
18. *The Guardian*, 26 February 2021.
19. Charteris-Black, J. (2019) *Metaphors of Brexit: No cherries on the cake?* London: Palgrave, Chapter 6.
20. https://www.ft.com/content/38a81588-6508-11ea-b3f3-fe4680ea68b5.
21. *The Independent*, 13 March 2020.
22. https://2sjjwunnql41ia7ki31qqub1-wpengine.netdna-ssl.com/wp-content/uploads/2021/01/MHP_Public-Poll-Covid-Terms_Tables_20-01-21.pdf. Accessed 24 June 2021.
23. *The Independent*, 24 March 2020.
24. *The Guardian*, 30 July 2020.
25. https://www.english-corpora.org/corona/.
26. *The Independent*, 4 December 2020.
27. *The Guardian*, 3 December 2020.
28. *Daily Mirror*, 30 December 2020.
29. *The Guardian*, 19 January 2021.
30. *The Guardian*, 6 January 2021.
31. Semantic prosody is the "consistent aura of meaning with which a form is imbued by its collocates". Louw, B. (1993) Irony in the Text or Insincerity in the Writer?—The Diagnostic Potential of Semantic Prosodies. In M. Baker, G. Francis & E. Tognini-Bonelli (eds.) *Text & Technology: In Honour of John Sinclair*. Amsterdam: Benjamins. P. 157.
32. **MAG**: America.
33. https://www.freep.com/story/news/politics/elections/2020/09/15/herd-mentality-trump-again-asserts-coronavirus-disappear/5812463002/. Accessed 24 June 2021.
34. *MailOnline*, 14 March 2020.
35. *telegraph.co.uk*, 2 March 2020.
36. *The Times*, 10 March 2020.
37. *The Independent*, 12 March 2020.
38. *The Times*, 13 March 2020.
39. *The Guardian*, 16 March 2020.
40. *MailOnline*, 16 September 2020.

41. https://www.ofcom.org.uk/__data/assets/pdf_file/0010/200503/media-nations-2020-uk-report.pdf. Accessed 24 June 2021.
42. i-*Independent Print Ltd*, 29 April 2014.
43. *The Daily Telegraph*, 10 October 2014.
44. https://www.english-corpora.org/corona/.
45. https://www.bbc.co.uk/news/uk-54255898. Accessed 24 June 2021.
46. *MailOnline*, 16 March 2020.
47. *Express Online*, 23 October 2020.
48. *The Times*, 9 January 1988.
49. *THE DAILY TELEGRAPH*, 25 February2003.
50. *Daily Mail*, 4 July 2007.
51. *The Guardian*, 31 July 2009.
52. *The Sunday Telegraph*, 25 September 2011.
53. *The Guardian*, 24 May 2015.
54. *The Guardian*, 26 October 2015.
55. *The Guardian*, 1 December 2014.
56. *Express Online*, 23 October 2020.
57. *The Daily Telegraph*, 19 September 2020.
58. *Daily Star Online*, 19 October 2020.
59. *telegraph.co.uk*, 9 April 2020.
60. Speech in Singapore parliament 23 February 1977.
61. Lee Kuan Yew Speech at the joint meeting of the United Nations congress 9 October 1985.
62. *The Guardian*, 18 September 2020.
63. *The Guardian*, 13 October 2020.
64. *The Guardian*, 14 October 2020.

6

Disease, Confinement and Language

Introduction

One way or another most people on the planet underwent some form of confinement during the period 2020–2021. Whether they were obliged to remain in their own room, stay in their flats or houses, obliged to stay within a specified distance from their home, or remain in their own region or country, the experience of reduced freedom of movement was universal. When outside, people were constrained by having to place a mask over their mouth and nose and, in some occupations, wear various forms of protective garment. Physical confinement was articulated through the concept of 'containment'. On March 3rd 2020, the UK government announced its four-pronged strategy: *contain*, delay, research and mitigate. The government declared that "The UK is currently focusing on *containing* the spread" and Matt Hancock, the Health and Social Care Secretary, announced: "We are taking all possible steps to *contain* this virus".

There was nothing new in ideas of containment and physical confinement during a pandemic. Throughout history the most common form of social response to the threat of infection has been control through confinement and I consider containment to be the abstract idea of confining a group of people within some form of bounded container. This could be by constructing separate physical spaces for those who are infected and by controlling the movement of those who are, or might be, infected between different geographical locations. In this chapter I consider the effect of the historical experience of disease-related confinement on cognition and on language by considering concepts such as 'quarantine' and the 'cordon sanitaire'. I trace historical implementation of containment policies by considering Daniel Defoe's *Journal of the Plague Year*, and the relationship between controlling disease and controlling crime. I also consider confinement as a form of treatment by looking at the 'iron lung'—a very special type of container that was used to treat polio patients. Part of the purpose of this is to demonstrate how moral frames are rooted in historical practice: relationships of Loyalty and Betrayal, Care and Harm, and Sanctity and Degradation have a degree of permanence in lived experience because of the historical context of confinement.

The last section examines how this historical experience of embodied confinement has contributed to the formation of conceptual categories for human cognition and their corresponding spatial metaphors. I discuss the 'container' schema and various conceptual metaphors that derive from this and how such spatial metaphors create models for understanding the constructs of the mind, the body, emotions, and the nation state. There is evidence in metaphor that all these are conceptually grounded in an abstract schema for containment.

The Cordon Sanitaire and the Pest House

In the absence of effective treatment, when threatened by highly infectious disease, the natural reaction of government has been to control its spread by the imposition and enforcement of boundaries—whether physical, bureaucratic or moral—around those who are believed to have the disease. Such boundaries, whether actual or abstract, are often referred to using a seventeenth century French term 'cordon sanitaire'. Linguistically, the 'cordon sanitaire' or 'line of health' is a spatial metaphor that works rather like the expression 'beyond the pale' where the 'Pale' was that part of Ireland where English rule prevailed; it was marked by a boundary on a map and 'pale' comes from the Latin *palum* a stake, and hence a fence. The cordon sanitaire is a conceptual and physically marked line that delineates a boundary patrolled by watchmen with the purpose of controlling the movement of people: it is a form of socially motivated container.

From the Middle Ages any person who had been in contact with an infected population was required to undergo a period of isolation, and from the time of the bubonic plague the term *quarantino* (40 days) refers to the period of time that was necessary for travellers to wait before they were permitted to leave the cordon sanitaire. From the fourteenth century cities around the Mediterranean including Ragusa (modern day Dubrovnik in Croatia), Marseilles, Venice, Pisa and Genoa imposed periods of quarantine. The choice of 40 days was probably motivated by the duration of Jesus's stay in the wilderness (subsequently commemorated by Lent), or other religious events such as the Flood. The word 'quarantine' is a metonym in which a number represents the period of time of enforced isolation. Such separation could be viewed either as a necessary precautionary measure to ensure public safety or as a form of group imprisonment, not one that was imposed for an act of crime but one necessary to prevent the transmission of disease.

In designing measures such as the quarantine there has always been tension between the medical exigency of preventing infection from spreading and the desire for freedom of those confined within, or contained by, the cordon sanitaire. Risk averse people prefer confinement measures, while less risk averse individuals place more emphasis on individual freedom and less on confinement. We saw this variation in the empirical research described in Chaps. 2 and 3. From the perspective of those not yet infected, the cordon was a necessary and rational form of protection, just like wearing clothes in cold weather. But from the point of view of those confined within the cordon, the barrier that separated them from others could be viewed as both restricting their liberty while simultaneously increasing the likelihood of their catching the disease by confining them to the company of the infected.

Infectious disease drives boundaries between people in different ways: it creates a division between the sick and the healthy, the infected and the uninfected, between those with knowledge—experts, epidemiologists, statisticians, doctors etc.—and those without specialist knowledge, between those who make the rules and those who are required to follow them. It also creates divisions among those with knowledge, for example in the coronavirus pandemic two contrary approaches, both supported by different groups of experts, have evolved: the lower risk option is containing the infection through a series of Lockdowns, this gives primacy to epidemiology while the higher risk approach holds that the majority should go about their daily lives as normal with voluntary confinement of the vulnerable, this gives primacy to economics and some mental health experts. This more libertarian approach takes a broader view of health including mental health and health conditions other than Covid-19 and is embodied in the Great Barrington Declaration.[1]

Historically, language has always played a crucial role in determining different perspectives on containment. Sometimes disease was prevented from entering or spreading within a town or village by constructing a 'pest house' away from the population. The term 'pest' originated from the French 'peste' meaning plague as this had been entering the country from the time of the Black Death onwards, the naming of illnesses usually points towards their foreign origin—whether it's the 'Spanish flu' (which originated in the United States), the 'British mutation of Covid-19',[2] the 'Kent' or the 'Indian' variant.[3] In the early fourteenth century, buildings for the isolation of those suffering leprosy were called *lazarettos*. Originating from the Nazareto quarantine station on an island off Venice, these buildings were constructed away from the population and the name *lazzaretto* was a blend of 'Nazareto' with 'Lazzaro', the Biblical figure of Lazarus who had become the patron saint of lepers in Catholicism.[4] Giving victims of the disease a connection with a religious saint invited compliance.

The influence of both metaphor and metonymy may determine whether the experience of confinement is perceived as enforced imprisonment, or as an act of self-imposed responsibility for the protection of society; the concept of 'confinement' implies that both are possible; for example, in the Coronavirus Corpus 'confinement' collocates with words such as 'forced' and 'mandatory' but also with 'voluntary'. In moral terms prison was primarily a form of punishment based on Fairness and Cheating, and only secondarily a form of protection of society by deterrence based on the moral foundation of Care and Harm. So, the purpose of protecting society was subservient to the moral intuition of giving the criminal the treatment they deserved. By contrast, the confined space of quarantine, in the pest house or lazaretto, although prison-like, had the primary purpose of protecting society hence the saintly name 'lazaretto'. Moral considerations also entered the equation if the disease itself had been contracted by inappropriate behaviours: sexually transmitted diseases were associated with prostitution or excessive lust. However, since the physical constraints were similar, the experience of imprisonment could metaphorically be transferred to that of quarantine as it was another form of enforced confinement. Public communication during times of pandemic is likely to emphasise that confinement is self-imposed and for the protection of 'loved ones' rather than a form of social imprisonment. This can be summarised conceptually by the contrast between CONFINEMENT IS IMPRISONMENT (as implied by the Great Barrington Declaration) and CONFINEMENT IS PUBLIC SAFETY (for example when the UK government policy introduced fines of £5000 for anyone travelling overseas without a defined reason).

Quarantine and Plague in the Seventeenth Century

The word quarantine comes specifically from *quaranta giorni*, meaning "forty days", in the Venetian language of the fourteenth and fifteenth centuries. As we saw above, during the period of plague known as the Black Death, this referred to the length of time for which all ships were required to be isolated before passengers and crew were allowed ashore. The most remarkable case of self-imposed confinement took place in 1665 when an outbreak of bubonic plague had spread from London to the small village of Eyam in the English Peak District. A complete cordon sanitaire was imposed under the leadership of the local young rector, William Mompesson, who provided a source of spiritual guidance throughout the duration of the plague in Eyam. This is summarised by Dr Michael Mosley in the following account published in the *Mail on Sunday* at the start of the pandemic in the UK:

A tailor from London arrived in the village of Eyam, population 380. He had with him samples of cloth. But the cloth also contained rat fleas, infected with bubonic plague. The records say he was bitten. But he made nothing of it, because at that time no one made any connection between plague and fleas. A few days later he died. Soon others started to die. Panic set in....

Those people who could afford to, fled. The squire and the landed gentry left within days, as did the local doctor. So the role of leader and hero fell to the young rector, 28-year-old William Mompesson. He called a town meeting and set in motion events that would ensure Eyam's place in history. First, they agreed there would be no more organised funerals or burials. People would have to bury their dead in local fields and gardens. Second, realising that the plague was contagious, they agreed that the church should be locked and all services held outdoors. It was believed that the minimum safe distance from someone contagious was 12 ft, which was actually about right. The third and hardest decision was to impose a 'cordon sanitaire' around the village—they would all go into self-isolation so as not to spread the plague to other communities. ... By November 1666, more than a year after it started, the plague had run its course...

Mompesson gathered them together and organised a mass burning to destroy anything that held 'the plague seeds'. As an example, he burnt everything he owned apart from the clothes he stood up in. By the time Christmas 1666 came around, people began to return and children were once again playing in the streets. This was to be the last outbreak of the Black Death in Britain. After nearly 300 years of constant eruptions, for no discernible reason it just died out.[5]

The village developed a system of obtaining supplies by leaving money in hollowed stones on the line of the cordon sanitaire, these was filled with vinegar as a disinfectant and supplies were left in return. What is remarkable in the account we have of Eyam is the proactive moral leadership at the local level, as summarised by a Victorian local historian William Wood:

Let all who tread the green fields of Eyam remember, with feelings of awe and veneration, that beneath their feet repose the ashes of those moral heroes, who with a sublime, heroic and unparalleled resolution gave up their lives, yea doomed themselves to pestilential death to save the surrounding country. Their self-sacrifice is unequalled in the annals of the world.[6]

Practices developed at Eyam formed the basis for later ideas such as Florence Nightingale's use of physical isolation to prevent infection from spreading at the time of the Crimean War, and the concept of the cordon sanitaire has continued up to the present with hospital isolation wards for patients being treated for Covid-19. Evidence of the relevance of this historical illustration of moral authority in times of pandemic is that there are 60 separate reports in which reference is made to 'Eyam' in the UK national press during the period 1st March 2020 to 1st March 2021; there are also 42 reports that make some reference to 'Cordon Sanitaire'.

Mompesson was only able to succeed in enforcing quarantine measures by substituting the frame of CONFINEMENT AS IMPRISONMENT with the frame of CONTAINMENT AS SPIRITUAL NECESSITY. By contrast, this was not always the case during the experience of the Great Plague of this time in London. There is a detailed and thorough account by Daniel Defoe in his *Journal of the Plague Year* when he describes the practice of enforced 'shutting up of house':

> This shutting up of houses was a method first taken, as I understand, in the plague which happened in 1603, at the coming of King James the First to the crown; and the power of shutting people up in their own houses was granted by Act of Parliament, entitled, 'An Act for the charitable Relief and Ordering of Persons infected with the Plague'.

And then refers to the new role of quarantine assessors in an Act of Parliament passed in July 1665:

The Examiner's Office

> That these examiners he sworn by the aldermen to inquire and learn from time to time what houses in every parish be visited, and what persons be sick, and of what diseases, as near as they can inform themselves; and upon doubt in that case, to command restraint of access until it appear what the disease shall prove. And if they find any person sick of the infection, to give order to the constable that the house be shut up; and if the constable shall be found remiss or negligent, to give present notice thereof to the alderman of the ward.

Houses that were suspected of containing a plague victim were put under 24-hour watch by the enforcers of quarantine—specially appointed watchmen:

Watchmen

That to every infected house there be appointed two watchmen, one for every day, and the other for the night; and that these watchmen have a special care that no person go in or out of such infected houses whereof they have the charge, upon pain of severe punishment. And the said watchmen to do such further offices as the sick house shall need and require: and if the watchman be sent upon any business, to lock up the house and take the key with him; and the watchman by day to attend until ten of the clock at night, and the watchman by night until six in the morning.

These measures are similar to those employed in China in the current pandemic:

Initially people were allowed out of their homes, but restrictions soon tightened. Some areas limited outings to one family member every two days to buy necessities. Others barred residents from leaving, requiring them to order in food and other supplies from couriers.

Later the policy became even more aggressive, with officials going door to door for health checks, and forcing anyone ill into isolation. A disabled boy reportedly died after he was left without food, water or help when his father and brother were quarantined.[7]

In 17th century London clearly defined laws covered every aspect of infectivity:

Sequestration of the Sick

As soon as any man shall be found by this examiner, chirurgeon, or searcher to be sick of the plague, he shall the same night be sequestered in the same house; and in case he be so sequestered, then though he afterwards die not, the house wherein he sickened should be shut up for a month, after the use of the due preservatives taken by the rest.

Airing the Stuff

For sequestration of the goods and stuff of the infection, their bedding and apparel and hangings of chambers must be well aired with fire and such perfumes as are requisite within the infected house before they be taken again to use. This to be done by the appointment of an examiner.

Shutting up of the House

If any person shall have visited any man known to be infected of the plague, or entered willingly into any known infected house, being not allowed, the house wherein he inhabiteth shall be shut up for certain days by the examiner's direction.

Every visited House to be marked

That every house visited be marked with a red cross of a foot long in the middle of the door, evident to be seen, and with these usual printed words, that is to say, "Lord, have mercy upon us," to be set close over the same cross, there to continue until lawful opening of the same house.

Watchmen were required to observe the marked house for 4 weeks to identify whether there were any plague cases. In seventeenth century London, there were clearly defined laws for the identification of disease and control of infection through confinement and other containment policies. The absence of any effective treatment for the plague placed even greater onus on the authorities to impose draconian measures that emphasised the need for physical separation of the infected. There was even an earlier form of 'social distancing' for those who came into contact with the infected:

That precise order to be taken that the searchers, chirurgeons, keepers, and buriers are not to pass the streets without holding a red rod or wand of three feet in length in their hands, open and evident to be seen, and are not to go into any other house than into their own, or into that whereunto they are directed or sent for; but to forbear and abstain from company, especially when they have been lately used in any such business or attendance.

Here the use of a 'wand of three foot in length' makes it clear that these are rules about PHYSICAL distancing, rather than 'social distancing'. The term 'social distancing' was a metonym because people were not supposed to avoid social contact as for example in online communication, but to keep apart when physically meeting others.[8] The metonym seems to be based on the idea that the physical body stands for the whole person. I have heard of walkers using walking sticks and those with impaired vision employing sticks for similar purposes during the current coronavirus pandemic. In some cases, the agents of government enforcement became the targets of physical assault that put their lives at risk:

> There was likewise violence used with the watchmen, as was reported, in abundance of places; and I believe that from the beginning of the visitation to the end, there was not less than eighteen or twenty of them killed, or so wounded as to be taken up for dead, which was supposed to be done by the people in the infected houses which were shut up, and where they attempted to come out and were opposed.

Defoe also makes an explicit connection between 'shutting up' houses and prisons, but also explains that they were not very effective prisons:

> Nor, indeed, could less be expected, for here were so many prisons in the town as there were houses shut up; and as the people shut up or imprisoned so were guilty of no crime, only shut up because miserable, it was really the more intolerable to them.
>
> It had also this difference, that every prison, as we may call it, had but one jailer, and as he had the whole house to guard, and that many houses were so situated as that they had several ways out, some more, some less, and some into several streets, it was impossible for one man so to guard all the passages as to prevent the escape of people made desperate by the fright of their circumstances, by the resentment of their usage, or by the raging of the distemper itself; so that they would talk to the watchman on one side of the house, while the family made their escape at another.

Without compliance and with their livelihoods at risk, then, as now, those who believed themselves to be wrongfully imprisoned, or those who had financial needs, took measures to obtain their liberty irrespective of the dangers to others, their own survival being a higher priority. He continues with the theme of ineffective prisons:

> It is to be considered, too, that as these were prisons without bars and bolts, which our common prisons are furnished with, so the people let themselves down out of their windows, even in the face of the watchman, bringing swords or pistols in their hands, and threatening the poor wretch to shoot him if he stirred or called for help.

In other cases, some had gardens, and walls or pales, between them and their neighbours, or yards and back-houses; and these, by friendship and entreaties, would get leave to get over those walls or pales, and so go out at their neighbours' doors; or, by giving money to their servants, get them to let them through in the night; so that in short, the shutting up of houses was in no wise to be depended upon. Neither did it answer the end at all, serving more to make the people desperate, and drive them to such extremities as that they would break out at all adventures.

The moral foundation of Liberty has often historically conflicted with Oppression and the resulting onus to subvert authority. He also comments on the inefficiencies of the system in noting the time lag between identification of an early symptom of infection and a response by the authorities; during this window of time, fearing enforced containment, those infected might spread the disease to those who were offering to assist them:

> In this interval, between their being taken sick and the examiners coming, the master of the house had leisure and liberty to remove himself or all his family, if he knew whither to go, and many did so. But the great disaster was that many did thus after they were really infected themselves, and so carried the disease into the houses of those who were so hospitable as to receive them; which, it must be confessed, was very cruel and ungrateful.

In the absence of symptoms nobody can be certain that they are not infected: we might *feel* perfectly well but nonetheless be the inadvertent transmitter of disease and only find out when it is too late. What has become known as the 'superspreader' may not even know that he or she is ill in the first place.[9] For those who did not have a safe place to go to outside of the city Defoe notes that some were successful by going into a form of self-imposed quarantine:

> ...other houses, where they locked themselves up and kept hid till the plague was over; and many families, foreseeing the approach of the distemper, laid up stores of provisions sufficient for their whole families, and shut themselves up, and that so entirely that they were neither seen or heard of till the infection was quite ceased, and then came abroad sound and well.

Overall, Defoe is critical of the prevention measures taken by the authorities because they treated the infected as criminals by imprisoning them in their own homes. As he notes, policies that prioritize confinement can have the opposite of their intended effect by pushing people to flee and spread the infection more widely:

> This is one of the reasons why I believed then, and do believe still, that the shutting up houses thus by force, and restraining, or rather imprisoning, people in their own houses, as I said above, was of little or no service in the whole. Nay, I am of opinion it was rather hurtful, having forced those desperate people to wander abroad with the plague upon them, who would otherwise have died quietly in their beds.

This is a point he reiterates:

> But, on the other hand, this was another of the inconveniences of shutting up houses; for the apprehensions and terror of being shut up made many run away with the rest of the family, who, though it was not publicly known, and they were not quite sick, had yet the distemper upon them; and who, by having an uninterrupted liberty to go about, but being obliged still to conceal their circumstances, or perhaps not knowing it themselves, gave the distemper to others, and spread the infection in a dreadful manner, as I shall explain further hereafter.

His view reflects the same tensions between the moral frames of Care/ Harm and Liberty/ Oppression that were noted earlier in this chapter in the discussion of the Great Barrington Declaration. Underlying the trope of confinement is, then, a concept in which the victims of illness are viewed as if they were prisoners, and while there are some correspondences between illness and crime, the two domains of experience are not always well mapped onto each other as illustrated in Fig. 6.1:

From Defoe's perspective on these two domains, it is only number six that appears to have any moral basis, numbers 1–5 have no moral basis, since crime is viewed as some form of intentional behaviour worthy of moral judgement, whereas this is rarely the case with disease, even 'superspreaders' may not be aware that they are such, and number 7 is named as having the contrary effect to that which was intended. There is some basis in this cognitive mapping that supports Defoe's negative evaluation

DOMAIN OF CRIME	DOMAIN OF DISEASE
1. CRIME	INFECTIOUS DISEASE
2. CRIMINAL	VICTIM, OR SPREADER OF AN
	INFECTIOUS DISEASE
3. TRIAL	MEDICAL EXAMINATION
4. VERDICT	DIAGNOSIS
5. IMPRISONMENT	ENFORCED QUARANTINE
6. INTENTION: STOPPING CRIME	INTENTION: STOPPING DISEASE
7. UNINTENDED CONSEQUENCE:	UNINTENDED CONSEQUENCE:
SPREADING CRIME	SPREADING DISEASE
8. PRISON WARDENS	WATCHMEN

Fig. 6.1 Mapping of 'crime' and 'disease'

of the practice of shutting people up in their houses. A typical example of deficiencies in the moral reasoning is that those responsible for enforcing confinement of the infected themselves became viewed as illegitimate sources of authority and became, sometimes justifiably, the target of abuse:

> sometimes the insolence, of the watchmen placed at their doors, those watchmen would answer saucily enough, and perhaps be apt to affront the people who were in the street talking to the said families; for which, or for their ill-treatment of the families, I think seven or eight of them in several places were killed; I know not whether I should say murdered or not, because I cannot enter into the particular cases.

Putting people under 'house arrest' for the benefit of the whole community was not something that is generally accepted in western democracies, although it is in China. But, as Defoe notes, it was based on mapping no. 6 the intention behind the measure:

> But after all that was or could be done in these cases, the shutting up of houses, so as to confine those that were well with those that were sick, had very great inconveniences in it, and some that were very tragical, and which merited to have been considered if there had been room for it. But it was

authorised by a law, it had the public good in view as the end chiefly aimed at, and all the private injuries that were done by the putting it in execution must be put to the account of the public benefit.

This conflict between desire for individual liberty and the risk this entails for others is one that characterises policies during the Covid-19 Pandemic, as we have already seen in disputes between supporters and opponents of the Great Barrington Declaration. People's personal freedoms—whether to go or not, to meet whom they want, or not, to wear a mask or not, to have a vaccine or not, to remain within their own home, region, country, or not—form the basis of their worldview. Using Haidt's moral foundations framework the frame of Care/ Harm—the desire to protect others—especially those who are vulnerable—is in conflict with the foundation of Liberty/ Oppression. It is for this reason that highly visible practices such as mask-wearing have become metonyms for ideological affiliation. The wearing of masks displays prioritisation of the moral foundation of Care/ Harm, whereas for anti-maskers the mask stands ideologically for Oppression. Removing 'the muzzle' places Liberty/ Oppression above the Care/ Harm moral foundation and became associated in the US with some Republican supporters of Donald Trump. By contrast, those who wore masks affiliated themselves with the Democratic party and other more left leaning outlooks that placed the moral foundation of Care/ Harm above that of Liberty/ Oppression.

It seems that when reflecting on seventeenth century London,[10] Defoe acknowledged the necessity of some confinement of the infected because of the dangers of not doing so and therefore accepted the Care/ Harm principle. But, overall, he is doubtful of the effectiveness of containment measures even when they are compliant with the moral authority of those who benefit from enforced confinement policies, because they are ineffective and impossible to enforce except on the poor:

> These things made it very hard, if not impossible, as I have said, to prevent the spreading of an infection by the shutting up of houses—unless the people would think the shutting of their houses no grievance, and be so willing to have it done as that they would give notice duly and faithfully to the magistrates of their being infected as soon as it was known by them-

selves; but as that cannot be expected from them, and the examiners cannot be supposed, as above, to go into their houses to visit and search, all the good of shutting up houses will be defeated, and few houses will be shut up in time, except those of the poor, who cannot conceal it, and of some people who will be discovered by the terror and consternation which the things put them into.

It seems quite possible that the same sort of considerations of how likely it is that citizens are to comply with restrictions placed on their liberty has determined a great deal of public policy communication in western democracies during the pandemic. The emphasis has been on providing information: the daily updates on cases, infection rates, and deaths—providing testing amenities and then, once available, a vaccination. While people are prepared to accept some limitations on their movements and contacts, they are less likely to comply with stringent measures such as complete lockdowns that are enforced with the full battery of State powers, except in non-western societies that have a tradition of state Authority. In western democracies, the emphasis has been on persuasion, rhetoric, information, and expert advice, rather than on rigid enforcement. The legal framework provides opportunities for fining those who infringe laws on social distancing, mask wearing etc. but these are only occasionally resorted to and only in more extreme cases of infringement. There is, then, a long history of the imposition of constraints on the movement of people, containment policies, and the use of confinement for disease control, especially in the absence of treatment measures. Linguistically, this has become embodied by the concepts of 'cordon sanitaire' and 'quarantine' and lexicalised concepts for social responses to infection control such as the 'social distancing' metaphor.

The Iron Lung

The social response to infectious disease has usually been to contain its spread by placing restrictions on the movement of bodies by confining them to ships, pest houses, the home or isolation wards. But historically, some virus symptoms have also demanded confinement of the patient's body, as when polio risks attacking the muscles of the chest and paralysing the diaphragm. One such treatment was the 'iron lung'—a type of container that could enable the body to respirate and prevent death by asphyxiation. Early forms of the iron lung resembled a large bellows, and the device itself was a mechanical substitution for natural respiration: the work of inhalation and exhalation that would normally be done by the contraction and expansion of the diaphragm is done by a body-sized cylinder, within which the patient is contained. The cylinder creates changes in air pressure around the body (which is why the body needs to be situated within the cylinder) forcing the patient's chest and abdomen to expand and contract exactly as a diaphragm would. A report from *The Independent* described a particular type of 'iron lung' as follows:

> The exovent uses the same principle as the old iron lungs by creating a negative pressure vacuum around the patient which gently forces air to be sucked into the lungs. It can be used to support patients to breathe or it can take over their breathing completely. Because the device fits over the patient on a hospital bed, they don't need to be sedated and can remain awake, eating and drinking and talking.[11]

Developed originally in the 1930s, and used more extensively during the polio epidemics of the 1940s and 50s, awareness of the iron lung was revived during the Covid-19 outbreak because of the shortage of ventilators. In spite of its associations with an earlier historical period some patients were still using an 'iron lung' in the twenty-first century and its principles were still deemed to be relevant as a form of treatment:

> The only treatment for those patients was to be placed into a 'iron lung', where they may have to stay for weeks, months or even years. Paul Alexander, a 74-year-old from Texas, caught polio in 1952 aged four and had to be put into an iron lung where he remains to this day.[12]

The Guardian interviewed Paul Alexander:

> The man in the iron lung When he was six, Paul Alexander was paralysed for life by polio. At 74, he's one of the last people alive still using an iron

lung. He sees parallels with his own experience in the Covid-19 pandemic, he tells Linda Rodriguez McRobbie. "It's exactly the way it was, it's almost freaky to me."[13]

The image of the iron lung—most of the body contained within a large metal cylinder and the patient's head protruding from an aperture at one end, potentially for very long periods of time—became a metaphor for enforced confinement during the Covid-19 pandemic. While victims were not forced into a cylinder, the sense of confinement could be *as if they were in an iron lung* but one that had the potential to save lives. Sometimes the 'iron lung' was used positively as a metaphor:

The housing market has been dubbed the economy's "iron lung"—but experts fear the boom will not last.[14]

In other cases, metaphors were used to describe the 'iron lung' as part of a moral warning to get vaccinated:

It may sound shocking to describe six weeks in hospital as a mild version of the illness, but this was a mysterious disease that paralysed and sometimes killed young children, leaving others unable to breathe without *an iron lung* which *entombed* their body.[15]

You have to be long in the tooth to recall poliomyelitis but it was a horrible *scourge*. It *stalked the halls* in my youth and when it *struck* it would *reduce* the sufferer to a life in *an iron lung* or at best a wheelchair.[16]

Here metaphor and metonymy is used as a powerful rhetorical tool to heighten the dangers of ignoring Covid-19 and therefore to endorse behaviours, such as vaccination, that resisted the spread of the disease. Because it was made of metal, the term 'iron lung' is also a double metonymy based on the material (iron) standing for the object and the function of an instrument standing for the function of a body part (the lungs). Sometimes metaphor could be a means for writers to comment on the wider political events of their times. With the onset of Covid-19 another literary classic that soon became a best seller was Albert Camus's *The*

Plague—often viewed as an allegory on the rise of Nazism. Although based on source material on the outbreak of cholera in Oran in 1849 (there were outbreaks of the plague in Oran in the twentieth century but they were small scale), the novel's appeal derived from the moral emphasis it replaced on the personal and social responses to the disease, especially the differing ways in which people react to the confinement required by the Cordon Sanitaire. Camus' daughter Catherine said: the message of the novel had newfound relevance in that "we are not responsible for coronavirus but we can be responsible in the way we respond to it".[17] So when commentators wanted to evaluate social and moral responses to Covid-19 they could either look back to medical history by drawing on the metonym of the iron lung, or they could comment more generally on confinement by using tropes derived from the works of writers such as Defoe and Camus.

Containment in Language

Given that the control of disease historically has entailed the construction of separate spaces to house the infected, and the confinement of people within their own houses for the protection of their community, it is not surprising that metaphors based on various forms of container have dominated much public discussion of the response to the Covid-19 pandemic. Words such as 'bubble', 'cocoon', 'pod', 'bunker', 'silo' and 'petri dish' dominated public communication and entered everyday language, at times even changing the language with the arrival of new verbs such as 'to bubble up with'. In this section I begin by considering some of the central ideas from cognitive linguistics related to schemas for 'containment' and illustrate how these have been taken up in the discourse of Covid-19 by examining their use in the UK press during a one-year period following the official acknowledgment of the disease in March 2020.

Lakoff and Johnson (1980) suggested that:

> We are physical beings. Bounded and set off from the rest of the world by the surface of our skins and we experience the rest of the world as outside us. Each of use in a container, with a bounding surface and an in-out ori-

entation. We project our own in-out orientation onto other physical objects that are bounded by surfaces. Thus we also view them as containers with an inside and an outside. ... But even where there is no natural physical boundary that can be viewed as defining a container, we impose boundaries-marking off territory so that it has an inside and a bounding surface-whether a wall, a fence, or an abstract line of plane. There are few human instincts more basic than territoriality. And such defining of a territory putting a boundary around it, is an act of quantification.[18]

The theory of embodiment that developed from this proposed that much of our thinking derived from experience of our bodies living within bounded spaces or, alternatively, experiencing our bodies as containers. Much of the evidence of claims for such 'image schemas' defined as "recurring, dynamic pattern[s] of perceptual interactions and motor programs that give coherence and structure to our experience" (Johnson 1987, p. xiv)." derived from prepositions such as 'into' or 'out of', especially when these did not refer to physical movements such as 'the ship is coming into view' or 'to fall in love'. Following this approach, the much-repeated slogan during the Coronavirus pandemic 'We are in all this together' is evidence of an image schema for containment.

The container schema is rather confusingly described by Lakoff and Johnson (1980) as an 'Ontological metaphor', confusingly because containment seems to be an embodied experience rather than a metaphor and this is better captured by the term 'schema' without proposing a more abstract level. They also proposed other spatial 'image schema', some of which are highly relevant to language and thought relating to the pandemic; these include 'source-path-goal' and 'centre-periphery'. The central argument of their seminal work is that our conceptual system is metaphorically structured and there was evidence for this in language. So, expressions such as 'I have had a full/ empty life' is evidence of a containment schema.[19] One of the difficulties in the pursuit of their main argument that the conceptual system is metaphorically structured is that using terms such as 'ontological metaphor' creates confusion since most definitions of metaphor assume a contrast with literal meaning. For a word or phrase to be a metaphor requires the possibility of the same word or phrase having another sense that is literal: there do not seem to be alternatives for expressions such as 'to fall in love', or even 'to be all in this together': is there any more embodied way of conveying this meaning? If not, though they are 'image schema' they are *not* necessarily metaphors. The confusion of 'image schema' with 'metaphor' has left terminological confusion as its legacy.

The Lakoff & Johnson interpretation of the container schema took its inspiration from the so-called 'Conduit metaphor' developed by Reddy (1973); this had proposed that language itself 'contained' meaning—'it's difficult to put into words', 'the meaning is in the words' or 'his words sounded hollow'. In this view, words are containers of meanings that are extracted from them when understanding their meaning. These quite abstract metaphors were expressed as:

TIME IS A CONTAINER	(Lakoff & Johnson 1980)
ARGUMENT IS A CONTAINER	(Lakoff & Johnson 1980)
LINGUISTIC EXPRESSIONS ARE	(Reddy 1973; Lakoff & Johnson
CONTAINERS FOR MEANING	1980)

In these an abstract entity is conceptualised as a container as, for example, in expressions such as 'just in time', 'your argument doesn't hold water' or 'it's difficult to put into words'. One important aspect of the schema for containment is its binary nature: something is either *in* or *out* of a container, just as with a prison, or a pest house, someone is either confined or not confined. This is important because metaphors derived from this schema carry with them the same binary nature. With infectious disease there are no half measures: the whole purpose of an isolation unit is defeated if there are any grey areas, and the rationale behind various controls on human behaviour is to enforce very clear divisions, a 'firewall', between what is within the container and what is outside the container. It is for this reason that containment schema are preferable to other schema such as 'source-path-goal or 'centre- periphery' since there are *degrees of* centrality or of distance. With 'journey' metaphors based on the source-path-goal schema, there are degrees of position along a path. For example, the name given by the British government to its policy to ending Lockdown was *'the roadmap"* and was announced on 17 May 2020:

Step-by-step unlocking: what happens when? *The roadmap* is underpinned by four key tests that are linked to data, which act like a checklist that must be met before moving on to the next step of reopening. The tests determine whether the vaccine rollout is going as planned; vaccines are effective in bringing down deaths and hospitalisations; case numbers are not rising so fast that the NHS risks being overwhelmed; and new variants do not create unforeseen risks.[20]

The concept of the roadmap dominated public communication of the ending of Lockdown and the metaphor of "the roadmap" referred to a series of events graded along a time-based path. This is not the case with the binary—'in'/'out'—nature of the containment schema because it was possible to measure progress along the correlation between what was allowed and a time sequence.

When we consider the importance of pandemic compliance there is no room for what became known in public discourse as 'mixed messaging'. This referred to a situation when people felt uncertain about how they were being required to behave by government. In their quest for clarity the government resorted to giving instructions that sought to eliminate uncertainty by strong sounding imperatives: 'Stay home, Protect the NHS, Save lives' which became replaced on 10th May 2020 with 'Stay Alert, Control the Virus, Save Lives'. This was one of a set of three-part slogans that included 'Catch it, Bin it, Kill it', 'Hands, Face, Space' and defined the rhetorical style of public communication during the pandemic. However, 'stay alert' referred to a mental state rather than a material one and was criticised for its lack of clarity. This is because it removed the containment schema implied by 'stay at home'.

Orientational metaphors based on the schema of motion from a source along a path towards a destination differ from the containment schema because they argue for *degrees of* progression. One can be at any unspecified position along a path in the right direction, so there is not the binary concept of being 'in' or 'out' implied by the containment schema. As part of its 'roadmap' the UK government used the metaphor of 'traffic lights' to set the rules for overseas travel. In May 2021 countries were classified as 'green', 'amber' or 'red' according to the level of quarantine they required on return. The same problem occurs with these tri-partite, 'traffic light' systems: they introduced a degree of confusion as many were unsure whether, or not, they were supposed to go to countries allocated an 'amber' status (such as most of the European Union).[21] There are two different strategies employed by drivers approaching an amber light: some prepare to stop for the anticipated red light, others put their foot down to get through the light before it turns red. Binary concepts are preferable for behavioural responses to viruses because there is less risk of confusion.

The centre-periphery schema applied in several ways during the pandemic. For example, it could refer to the distance from the centre of an infection as in the following:

On 22 March, Mayor Bill de Blasio called New York City the epicentre of the coronavirus crisis. The state has the most cases in the US, and the city has the most cases in the state. Queens, the borough in which I live, has had the most deaths in the city, and Elmhurst Hospital—which at times has been operating at more than 100 per cent capacity—is about 1 mile away from my apartment. Call this the epicentre of the epicentre of the epicentre.[22]

Here the writer is gauging his safety with a metaphor based on the relative proximity of his apartment to the area where coronavirus was at its most virulent. The word 'epicenter' collocates with disease related words such as 'outbreak', 'deadly' and 'crisis' implying a high level of danger. Government responses such as testing, and vaccination were directed towards such 'epicentres' and in some cases there were local Lockdowns based on degrees of proximity to these 'centres' of the infection. In practice, though, a linear concept became a binary one, as the actual zones of local Lockdowns were based on administrative frontiers that served as cordons sanitaire. The center-periphery schema also applied in relation to social distancing in terms of deciding how close people could be physically, especially when public messaging apps could indicate to customers of bars and restaurants how near they had been to an infected person, and therefore whether they needed to get tested or go into quarantine. So the 'centre' of this schema could either be a geographical area or an infected body and degrees of safety were then measured in terms of distance from this area of body.

At times there was a confusion in public messaging because of a tension between the medical need to prevent infection from spreading by keeping people within confined spaces, or zones and, the less mandatory phrasing that appears more socially acceptable within democracies. The more flexible schema of source-path-destination (e.g. 'the roadmap', 'traffic lights)' was attractive to politicians because they did not imply fixed points of measurement but were much less effective when applied to public health related behaviour. There was a rhetorical need for public messaging to distance itself from the associations of the 'pest house' or the 'leper colony' by creating types of metaphoric container that would be attractive for people to enter and remain within: these sorts of container were best communicated by metaphors that had positive associations such as protection, amusement and nature, this is where the metaphors of 'the bubble' and 'the cocoon' entered the language.

Much previous research into metaphor that has applied the containment schema has derived from psychology rather than from the social sciences. Evidence from idioms suggested underlying conceptualisations of the body, or parts of the body, as a container that provided evidence for conceptual metaphors; for example:

> …the idiomatic expression "John spilled the beans" maps our knowledge of someone tipping over a container of beans to that of a person revealing some previously hidden secret. English speakers understand "spill the beans" to mean "reveal the secret" because there are underlying conceptual metaphors, such as THE MIND IS A CONTAINER and IDEAS ARE PHYSICAL ENTITIES, that structure their conceptions of minds, secrets, and disclosure. (Gibbs 2019, p. 40)

Idioms related to emotions such as 'contain yourself', 'making one's blood boil', or 'simmer down' implied a conceptual metaphor THE BODY IS A CONTAINER FOR THE EMOTIONS and derived from various other conceptual metaphors such as ANGER IS HOT FLUID IN A CONTAINER (Gibbs 1990), and the more general EMOTIONS ARE FLUIDS IN A CONTAINER. While there is much debate over the reality of these conceptual metaphors, what is worth noting is that these are ways of expressing affective states rather than public policy. So, somebody talking about children needing to 'let off steam' when they are released from classroom into a playground, or a couple who are 'blowing their lids', regularly because they are cooped up in the same house for much longer than usual is referring to the experience of Lockdown from the perspective of individual states of mind. The idea of the body as a container can be extended to particular body parts, as Illustrated by Ray Gibbs:

> One image schema that is frequently employed in metaphorical thought and language is CONTAINMENT. The CONTAINMENT image schema underlies many metaphorical concepts related to our understanding of linguistic action. For instance, our mouths, like our bodies, are experienced as containers, such that when the container is open, then linguistic action is possible, and when closed, there is only silence. To be "closed-lipped" reflects the silent, closed container, and when one "bites one's lip," the closing of the mouth and lips is done quickly with great force.

The following conceptual metaphors have been proposed in the literature:

MIND IS A CONTAINER	(Lakoff & Johnson 1980)
ANGER IS HOT FLUID IN A CONTAINER	(Gibbs 1990)
BODY IS A CONTAINER FOR THE EMOTIONS	(Kövecses 2003; Charteris-Black 2004)
EMOTION IS A SUBSTANCE IN A CONTAINER	(Kövecses 2003)

All of these can be subsumed under the more general conceptual metaphor THE BODY IS A CONTAINER. These were well established in language, especially in relation to the expression of human emotions through a range of words from the semantic field of liquids for emotion concepts as in 'waves' or 'surges', of emotion, 'undercurrents' of feeling, or pressures on the container—as in 'floods of tears', 'outbursts of anger', 'pouring out one's heart', 'gushing with emotion' etc. (Goatly 2007: 197ff.). Such expressions entail that the body is experienced as a container and the inherent instability of emotions may be traced to the association of emotion with changed states and loss of control as the forces that build up in a container pressurise its boundaries. These derive from embodied experience of pressure and the movement of blood within the body when intense emotions are experienced.

People became very aware of their mouths as possible containers of infection during the pandemic. The mouth and breathing organs became the focus of infection control, so that the act of covering the mouth with a mask became the most basic level of control, and since Covid-19 was spread by aerosol, the force with which an infected person sneezed or coughed influenced the extent to which those in the vicinity risked getting infected. Mouth covering became a central goal of public health communication, along with avoiding touching the face with unwashed hands. Here the mask became metonymically related to the mouth, so that the uncovered mouth was a metonym for infectivity, whereas a covered mouth became a metonym for control of infection. The body, and in particular the breathing organs and the mouth, were literally the container of the Covid-19 virus and the masked or unmasked mouth took on ideological meanings. Metonymy was evident in this literal act of mouth covering and the equally literal swab testing from the oral cavity, and this is discussed in Chap. 8, but the container schema remained implicit.

By contrast, metaphor was much more prevalent in social policy and political messaging in relation to containment of the body as, for example, when public communication exhorted people to 'stay within their social bubbles'. These metaphors were used to express *social* rather than personal experience and the following conceptual metaphors have been suggested:

BRITAIN IS A CONTAINER	(Charteris-Black 2006)
NATIONS ARE CONTAINERS	(Charteris-Black 2006)
BOUNDARIES ARE CONTAINERS	(Charteris-Black 2012, 2019)
CONTAINERS ARE BOUNDED SPACES	(Charteris-Black 2019)

In all these concepts the body is contained by an external entity and Chilton (2004)[23] argues convincingly for the importance and pervasiveness of these spatial metaphors in relation to political discourse. He proposes a container schema in which 'what is inside is close to the self, and what is outside is also outside the law'. He also refers to 'a spatial containment schema which grounds conceptualizations of one's country as a closed container that can be sealed or penetrated' (ibid.: 118). Chilton (1996) explained how the notion of 'containment' was used by the USA as a strategy for controlling the spread of Communism in Eastern Europe and how the Cuban missile crisis of 1961 was conceptualised as penetrating the American security sphere.[24] Historically, the notion of 'containment' applied much more frequently in relation to foreign rather than domestic policy decisions. If you could not prevent something at its source you could at least control the reach of its influence. There was therefore already a tradition for government policies to be communicated with metaphors based on the abstract schema of containment.

In a study of British immigration-related metaphors I proposed that the concept of a loss of control can be equated to the perforation of a container and penetration of a bounded area, hence in rhetorical terms loss of control arouses the emotion of fear of external dangers, like a hole in a mosquito net. The existence of a container implies both an inside and an outside and in relation to political discourse requires both the 'Us' and the 'Them' referred to by Van Dijk (ibid.); the penetration of the boundary of a container implies that the 'them' is symbolically entering the 'us'.[25] Metaphors of external containment such as 'bubbles' in which the body is experienced as the thing that is contained were much more predominant during the period of the pandemic because people were experiencing physical containment quite literally, they were therefore activated by the situational context. There is evidence of the schema for containment in the Prime Minister's address to the nation on 4th January 2021 which announced the nation's third national Lockdown:

> In England, we must therefore go *into* a national lockdown which is tough enough to contain this variant. That means the Government is once again instructing you to stay at home.

He had not used the expression '*into* a national lockdown' when announcing the first Lockdown of 23rd March 2020, but now the concept of a lockdown was an established one it could be conceptualised as a container.

Containment and control are therefore two very closely related and mutually supportive concepts that are closely related to confinement in policy formation during a pandemic.

Summary

Containment and confinement are embodied experiences that motivate many of the metaphors and metonyms during pandemics and provide the basis for understanding the relationship between the individual's body, language, and the body politic, the society. This becomes greatly accentuated in times of pandemic because there is a medical need to confine humans to particular locations. Following the rider of reason, the diseased body is placed within a designated structure: a house, a hospital, an intensive care unit and the possibly infected body is confined within actual or notional boundaries that impose limits on its movement. Confinement is an embodied experience that either can be imposed by external forces or selected by the individual and there is evidence of both these practices in Defoe's account of the plague. The container schema has been employed for interpreting various metaphors related to emotions, body parts, nations and their policies and can be employed for public communication during any pandemic. In the next chapter I explain how this schema accounts for a great deal of English language public communication during the Coronavirus epidemic that struck in 2020.

Notes

1. https://gbdeclaration.org/. Accessed 24 June 2021.
2. Angel Merkel, 22 March 2021: "We are now basically in a new pandemic. The British mutation has become dominant".
3. The naming of these diseases is discussed in Chap. 8.
4. https://www.sciencefriday.com/articles/the-origin-of-the-word-quarantine/. Accessed 24 June 2021.
5. *MailOnline*, 28 March 2020.
6. https://www.ool.co.uk/blog/what-part-did-eyam-play-against-the-plague/. Accessed 24 June 2021.
7. https://www.theguardian.com/world/2020/mar/19/chinas-coronavirus-lockdown-strategy-brutal-but-effective. Accessed 24 June 2021.

8. See Nerlich, B. and Jaspal, R. (2021). Social representations of 'social distancing' in responseto Covid-19 in the UK media. *Current Sociology*, 1–18. first online. https://doi.org/10.1177/0011392121990030.

9. The term 'superspreader' is discussed in Chap. 7 in the section entitled 'The petri-dish metaphor'.

10. Although it describes the events of 1665, the book was not published until 1722.

11. *The Independent*, 20 January 2021.

12. *MailOnline*, 16 December 2020.

13. *The Guardian*, 26 May 2020.

14. *The Express*, 8 October 2020.

15. *The Independent*, 23 August 2020.

16. *The Express*, 16 October 2020.

17. *The Guardian*, 28 March 2020.

18. Lakoff, G. and Johnson, M. (1980) *Metaphors We Live By*. Chicago, IL: University of Chicago Press, p. 29.

19. Most linguists now usually refer to 'schema' rather than 'image schema' and this is my practice in this book.

20. *telegraph.co.uk*, 14 June 2021.

21. The Labour Party argued against the 'amber' status.

22. *The Independent*, 16 April 2020.

23. Chilton, P. (2004) *Analysing Political Discourse*. London and New York: Routledge.

24. Chilton, P. (1996) *Security Metaphors: Cold War Discourse from Containment to Common House*. New York: Peter Lang.

25. The framing of 'invasion' as 'rape' is discussed in Lakoff, G. (1991).

7

'Bubbles', 'Cocoons', the 'Protective Ring' and the 'Petri Dish': The Containment Frame and the Pandemic

Introduction

Following the general discussion of historical ideas regarding confinement, in this chapter I discuss a series of dominant metaphors relating to a schema for containment and contributed to the public discourse of the pandemic; these include 'bubble', 'cocoon', 'protective ring' and 'petri dish'. I will refer to these as 'containment metaphors' and suggest that they had loosely defined rhetorical objectives such as creating social cohesion through articulating shared values and expressing moral intuitions. These included the need to protect the vulnerable from harm and to ensure the compliance by the majority with Lockdown rules through appealing to the intuitions of Loyalty and Fairness. However, I will also suggest that these metaphors were not always particularly Honest and can provide examples of the Dishonesty of official communication. I hope to illustrate the role of metaphors in debates around the public communication of pandemic policies and to describe the moral intuitions on which they were based.

Table 7.1 indicates the number of different stories in the UK Press classified under the theme of coronavirus over the one-year period from 1st March 2020 that referred to each of the container related terms discussed in this chapter:

© The Author(s), under exclusive license to Springer Nature Switzerland AG 2021
J. Charteris-Black, *Metaphors of Coronavirus*,
https://doi.org/10.1007/978-3-030-85106-4_7

Table 7.1 Containers in the UK Press (1 March 2020–28 February 2021)

Container	Number of stories
Bubble	10,000+
Pocket	7509
Bunker	1031
Cocoon	766
Pod	675
Petri dish	495
Protective ring	335
Fish bowl	75

In each section I illustrate a particular containment metaphor then explore its moral intuitions through a discussion of its linguistic characteristics by answering the following questions:

1. What is the container and what is contained?
2. Does the container protect, and if so from what?
3. Does the container restrict or constrain the entity contained?
4. What are the properties of the container?
5. What is the viewpoint? (From within or outside of the container).
6. What is the transitivity & agency of what is in the container and what puts them there?

The heuristics of these questions will hopefully provide insight into the cognitive structure, moral frames, and ideology of containment metaphors.

The 'Bubble' Metaphor

The most common containment metaphor was 'bubble' and it combined an appeal to the moral frame of Care with that of Loyalty by arguing that to care for society and protect others one had to be loyal to those who were 'in' one's own 'bubble'. In this section I describe some of the characteristics of the 'bubble' metaphor and point out some of its inadequacies. While the 'bubble' metaphor had the advantages of implying a flexible container, its usual meaning in English has been rather negative, something that implied detachment and a separation that was either transitory or harmful. Consider expressions like 'housing bubble', 'speculative bubble' or 'credit bubble' which imply something that is likely to end soon, or 'social media bubble', 'filter bubble' or 'intellectual bubble' which imply a type of intellectual detachment that is damaging:

> For example, in American Amusement Machine Association v. Kendrick, an appellate court held: "People are unlikely to become well-functioning, independent-minded adults and responsible citizens if they are raised in an intellectual bubble.".[1]

This sense of bubble is rather like the 'echo chamber' where lack of exposure to the views of others reinforces prejudice and confirms bias. It was therefore perhaps surprising that when Boris Johnson introduced his policy in a Statement on 10th June 2020 there were 17 instances of the metaphor 'bubble':

> From this weekend, we will allow single adult households—so adults living alone or single parents with children under 18—to form a *"support bubble"* with one other household.
>
> All those in a *support bubble* will be able to act as if they live in the same household—meaning they can spend time together inside each others' homes and do not need to stay 2 metres apart.

Without acknowledgment, he was adopting a metaphor that was first used by Jacinda Ardern, the Prime Minister of New Zealand, on 24th March 2020, and its motivation is described as follows:

> However, in her next daily briefing she floated another more specific metaphor. We heard her encourage us to, "stick to your bubble," and "you can't spend time with other people outside of your bubble".
>
> We are very familiar with the behaviour of bubbles: they froth on the ocean, they slide down the dishes, and they glide by on those summer afternoons when children form them with detergent and plastic hoops.
>
> The use of bubbles here conjures up an image of me and my loved ones floating around inside a transparent membrane that separates my group out from others and protects us from unwanted intrusion.[2]

Very soon a whole flurry of compound forms had evolved from this metaphor. I searched the UK national press database on Nexis for stories

Table 7.2 'Bubble' compound nouns (UK Press, 1 March 2020–28 February 2021)

Compound form	Example	Stories (N)[a]	Earliest use
Support bubble	There are only a few instances where it would be safe to visit this Mother's Day. As you are allowed to exercise and socialise outside with one other person (keeping your distance if you aren't part of the same household or *support bubble*), you could meet your mother for a walk, coffee or picnic if she lives close by.	3465	*telegraph. co.uk*, March 21, 2020
Social bubble	But, people should still avoid mingling beyond a small *social 'bubble'*, and work from home still if they can.	721	*The Guardian*, 27 April 2020
Travel bubble	Borders could soon be re-opened between Australia and New Zealand under a *'travel bubble'* scheme being discussed by Ms Ardern and Australian Prime Minister Scott Morrison.	533	*MailOnline*, 28 April 2020
Biosecure bubble	Now they face a new and completely unexpected test: Cramming a summer of international cricket into nine weeks at sterilised empty grounds and living life in a *biosecure bubble*.	393	*telegraph. co.uk*, 13 May 2020
Childcare bubble	Visiting those in your support bubble (or your *childcare bubble* for childcare);	265	*telegraph. co.uk*, 26 March 2020
Household bubble	Takeaway meals and food delivery would be allowed again and people could once again see partners who did not live with them, or bring an "exclusive" number of others, such a single person, relative or caregiver for their children into their *household "bubble"*.	173	*The Guardian*, 16 April 2020

[a]Nexis, Accessed 6 June 2021

that were classified under the theme 'Coronaviruses' to find the frequency of compound forms including 'bubble'. Table 7.2 shows the number of stories that included forms occurring in at least 100 stories and the earliest use of the metaphor:

When used literally a container is a physical object that has a clearly defined boundary, and when used as a metaphor it is something that does not physically contain but confines in some other way; for example, the expression 'travel bubble' provides a legal status for moving between only two countries. In Covid-19 policy statements the 'bubble' metaphor confined people to a social unit that had the purpose of preventing infection and the spread of the disease. The 'bubble' was supposed to provide a barrier that protected whoever was within it from the external virus and had the reciprocal role of protecting the social world outside the 'bubble' from any infection contained within it: it sought to appeal to the moral intuitions of Loyalty and Care and Harm as the bubble was not framed as restricting or constraining the people that it contained: this was a metaphor for an, apparently, voluntary confinement.

Considering question 4 (above), the bubble is transparent, but since one of its properties is fragility, it can easily be burst, as, say, in 'dot.com bubble' or 'tech bubble', but in its new Covid policy sense the fragility implied that people should act to maintain the integrity of their 'bubble' to avoid it being burst, in moral terms people had to be Loyal to their 'bubble'. What is worth noting is how the reciprocity implied by the 'bubble' complies with moral principles grounded in the idea that there is some form of balance between the reciprocal obligations of the individual towards their own group, or family, while at the same time protecting the outside society from what is within their family, so the 'bubble' metaphor appealed to the moral frame of Fairness. The nuclear family was probably better suited to this type of 'bubble'. For extended families with large numbers of different generations, the 'bubble' was inherently less protective since there was no escape permitted from it: Loyalty to the family 'bubble' was sometimes therefore paradoxically in conflict with Fairness as Covid-19 cases were higher in extended families and these were often from minority ethnic backgrounds.

An important aspect of a bubble is that its boundary is formed by a liquid and although liquids can be transparent, this is not always the case, for example bubble gum is opaque and even a clear bubble may refract the light creating a spectrum of colours, but a bubble generally permits the external viewer to see what is contained within. This was an important aspect of the 'bubble' metaphor from the point of view of public policy, because, like Bentham's Panoptican, it offered a covert form of social control as once outsiders knew who was within a 'bubble', they could notice any intruders into that 'bubble'. However, where the 'bubble' differed from the Panoptican was as regards viewpoint (question 5). The Panoptican was a system of observation by a prison guard who could survey all cells from a single point from within a circular prison, by contrast, with the 'bubble', the viewpoint was typically from *outside* as people talked about 'your' or 'their' bubble' more than they did 'my bubble'; this is illustrated in Table 7.3:

Table 7.3 shows that it was more common to use plural forms of pronouns ('our', 'their'), since typically a bubble contained several people, and that the second-person form ('your') and third-person form ('their') were both more common than either of the first-person forms ('my' and 'our'). The second- and third-person forms of pronouns imply an external perspective:

> You can expand this to connect with close family and whanau, bring in caregivers, or support isolated people. It's important to protect *your bubble*. Keep *your bubble* exclusive and only include people where it will keep you and them safe and healthy. If anyone within *your bubble* feels unwell, they legally must immediately self-isolate from everyone else within the bubble.[3]

> We're in a difficult period and I really do hope we see people are sensible and stay within their family or *their bubble* to stop the spread of this awful virus that has killed so many people.[4]

What this suggests as far as agency is concerned (question 6 above) is that 'bubble' was a concept related to social imposition of behaviours on others rather than being self-selected. While you were given the right to choose who was in your bubble it was an external force that required you

Table 7.3 Possessive pronouns and 'bubble' in the coronavirus corpus

	N
My bubble	181
His/ her bubble	102
Our bubble	336
Your bubble	880
Their bubble	557

to stay in that bubble. So, while the 'bubble' metaphor implied a light touch approach to social regulation, Johnson's exhortation to form a support bubble was a moral constraint on Liberty; however, this confinement was designed to appeal to the moral intuitions of Care, Loyalty, and Fairness.

Of course, 'bubble' was stylistically a very different metaphor from another prison related one—'Lockdown'; this had originated in the practice in the US of confining prisoners to their cells as punishment for acts of group disobedience. The metaphor broadened over time so that it became applied to a range of different social situations where constraints were placed on human movement. The implication of a 'Lockdown' is that there is an external force that exerts a downwards pressure on the entities within a contained space (i.e. the prisoners), by contrast, the fragility and expandability of a 'bubble' frames the decision to say in a confined space as one of *choice*, so it has some appeal to the frame of Liberty. However, both are forms of containment metaphor in so far as they prescribe limits on freedom of movement. As far as agency is concerned, in Lockdown agency derived from the *institution that enforces the lockdown*, whereas with 'bubble' there is a degree of *negotiated agency* so that it is less clear that there are a set of subject-object relations. One example of the persuasive effect of agency is that 'bubbles' were typically 'created':

> My family and I washed our hands constantly. We were careful about what we ate. For the most part, though, we just stayed home. They *created a bubble* around me, to protect me.[5]

> This is called making *a 'support bubble' and once created* you can think of yourself as being in a single household with people from the other household.[6]

The notion that a confined group of people was an act of *creation* attributes agency to those who are in the 'bubble' and implies that since they are involved in creating it, they are more likely to keep within it—as is fitting with voluntary confinement. It is therefore a use of language the exhorts a moral emotion based on reason. This contrasts with Defoe's observation noted in the last chapter that those who were required to remain within their houses by physical force, frequently sought to break out—as if from prison. Linguistic innovation occurred in 'bubbling' that became both an adjective:

> but the UK has endured arguably more dramatic events: the cancellation *Christmas bubbling* plans, followed by the temporary ban from many countries on travellers from the UK.[7]

And, more significantly, a verb with a human subject

> These rules will allow families to '*bubble*' *with* two other households in all four home nations between December 23 and 27, but those bubbles cannot meet inside pubs, hotels, shops, theatres or restaurants.[8]

> What if a family member tests positive while I'm *bubbled up*?[9]

Once people started to talk about 'to bubble with' or 'being bubbled up' the concept had become lexicalised.

In evaluating the 'bubble' metaphor while it has the advantage of inviting a degree of negotiation between agents, I have also noted that a common verb collocate of 'bubble' is 'burst' as in the financial contexts I have mentioned above such as 'speculative bubble'. 'Burst' is the second most frequent verb preceding 'bubble' in the BNC[10] and the ninth most frequent verb preceding 'bubble' in the Coronavirus Corpus. The 'bubble' metaphor has been used historically to describe financial speculation in expressions such as 'The South Sea Bubble'—bubbles whose volatility led to their bursting. This sense is evident in the following entry for 'bubble':

> Figurative use in reference to anything wanting firmness, substance, or permanence is from 1590s. Specifically in reference to inflated markets or financial schemes originally in **South Sea Bubble**, which originated c. 1711 and collapsed 1720.[11]

Surely qualities such as 'firmness' and 'permanence' are rather important in the management of a major pandemic? Unfortunately, a pandemic is not a bubble that can simply be burst, and so perhaps metaphors that required a higher degree of firmness about social interactions might have created conditions that were safer and less likely to contribute to further infection? If this is the case, then I raise doubts as to the effectiveness of the 17 'support bubble' metaphors in Boris Johnson's policy statement of 10th June 2020. As well as carrying rather negative ideas of detachment as in expressions such as 'the media bubble', or 'The Westminster bubble', the word carries with it ideas of triviality, ephemera and lack of substance—metaphors, some thought, for the Prime Minister himself.

The 'Cocoon' and 'Shielding' Metaphors

The British government had become aware of the importance of finding language that would encourage compliance with Covid-19 restrictions on public behaviour and often relied on metaphor to achieve this objective by appealing to the moral frame of Care. A central metaphor in its communication strategy was that of 'cocoon', that safe, womb-like space that allows a chrysalis to grow until it is ready to emerge in all its glory; the word occurred in 1,675 different stories in the British press ('cocoon', cocoons', 'cocooned' or 'cocooning') in the one-year period from 1st March 2020. It was sometimes used in expressions such as 'Lockdown cocoon' or 'love cocoon'.

On 29th June 2020 the government issued a document entitled "Guidance on cocooning to protect people over 70 years and those extremely medically vulnerable from COVID-19—updated guidance" that stated its policy for coming out of the Lockdown that had been in place since 23rd March 2020. This text demonstrated the first explicit integration of a containment metaphor into public policy during the crisis. 'Cocoon' was put forward as a concept to encourage the elderly to protect themselves from infection by staying indoors. 'Cocoon' occurs 30 times in the guidance, and it is worth looking at some of these. Linguistically, the document commenced with a broad definition of 'cocooning':

> *Cocooning* is a measure to protect people who are over 70 years of age and those who are extremely medically vulnerable…

It does not yet tell you what cocooning entails, but it indicates its purpose. It continues:

> *Cocooning* is advised for your personal protection and you will make your own judgement about the extent to which *cocooning* guidance applies to you. If you are unsure whether or not you fall into one of the categories of extremely medically vulnerable people listed above, you should discuss your concerns with your GP or hospital clinician.
>
> It is recognised that you have the right to exercise your own judgement as to the extent to which you consider the *cocooning* guidance appropriate for you. However, older people (aged 70 years and over) and those with pre-existing chronic conditions have been found to be more susceptible to COVID-19 infection and are most likely to experience severe consequences from infection so it is still recommended that you remain *cocooned* for your safety.

The wording here is a little contrary, it begins by acknowledging that interpretation is a matter of personal choice, a voluntary confinement, but then specifies the social groups for whom the guidance becomes 'recommended'. Notice that the contrastive 'however' in the second paragraph implies that these groups should *not* be exercising their personal judgement but following what is 'recommended'- and hence implies a more mandatory confinement; individual assessment of risk is therefore subservient to social categorization as 'older' or having 'chronic conditions'. Of course, once something was 'recommended' it not only limited the agency of older people but also jeopardised the position of their carers; once I heard these restrictions, I was much less keen to take my mother out in her wheelchair for her favourite 'walk' around the lake because it would now be my fault if anything went wrong. Had I known that she would not outlive the pandemic I might have done otherwise, but at the time the official message was that caution should override considerations of quality of life. Fortunately my mother was not always so cowed by official discourse.

What we should note in this government guidance is that 'cocooning' is used predominantly as a verb (underlined), as a form of social practice, and it is this theme that is developed:

> make the journey alone, with *someone who is cocooning* with you or at least someone who is in your core group of family or friends. You can also have

visitors to your home, ideally from the same core group of family or friends who are aware of your circumstances and willing to adhere to protective measures *while you cocoon*.

if you wish, you can indicate that *you are cocooning* to the service provider…

Whilst the rest of your household are not required to adopt these protective *cocooning measures* for themselves, we would expect them to do what they can to *support you in cocooning*…

The repetition of 'cocoon' as a verb indicates an intention by the authors to establish the concept so that it no longer just a metaphor but becomes embedded in social practice. The word 'cocoon' originates in the French *coucon* which is related to 'coque'—a clam shell, egg shell or nut shell. The concept of a shell carries with it associations of fragility; as with 'bubble', the idea of the container as fragile implies that great care is needed to protect it, both by those within it and others outside of it. As a metaphor it entails protection without excessive constraint, a self-selected action by whatever is contained within the cocoon, so it is nestles within the moral frame of Care, at least until it can emerge as part of a natural cycle.

Some commentators, such as Robert Fisk, were critical of the 'cocoon' concept seeing it as somewhat Orwellian:

I notice that this is beginning—in the case of the elderly—to morph into the idea of "cocooning", another suspicious expression which originally applied to insects. To act like an insect might be safer than membership of a herd but the idea of a cocoon in its new linguistic use implies a "wake-up" time which some of those sleeping away may not ultimately enjoy.[12]

He views 'cocooning' suspiciously on the grounds that those who are 'cocooned' might not desire the isolation and separation that it entailed because it was behaviour that one associates with insects rather than with humans and is, therefore, potentially dehumanising. Fisk also viewed the use of such containment metaphors as patronising:

Are most folk not mature enough to understand just plain "distancing" or even "health distancing" which is, after all, the point? Must the elderly be ridiculed by being told they must "cocoon", as if they are each to be turned into a chrysalis which may—or may not—awaken? Must we have "bubbles" for families and "pods" for children? However low the estimation of their people may be by members of the British cabinet, they do not have to treat their citizens as babies.

An infantilised society will not be able to imagine a new future; nor answer the demands of future generations of society of every origin which—far from being "distanced"—must be socially united.[13]

Is Fisk just being curmudgeonly or is the language of these metaphors fundamentally lacking in Honesty by patronizing people? Fisk was not alone in his criticism of the concept:

> The political philosopher Matthew Crawford is one of those who believes that western societies are being blighted by what he terms safetyism, the elevation of safety above all else. He argues that when the state cocoons its citizens from dangers, people lose the elemental pleasure, autonomy, mastery and sense of discovery that comes from taking their own decisions and risks. … I am with Crawford in thinking our culture underrates the downsides of security, and the inevitability and necessity of risk. I am for fire safety and seat belts but also for accepting that challenge and danger are an inescapable part of a full life.[14]

> *The Sunday Telegraph* warned: "PROLONGED periods of lockdown that *cocoon* the public from germs could leave people vulnerable to new viruses, a leading epidemiologist has warned."[15]

Such authors were concerned that having exhorted people to go into their cocoons they might not want to emerge from them again, after all, it is perfectly safe, snug and warm in a cocoon—especially one that is provided for by Amazon deliveries and good broadband connection. By encouraging an almost infantile dependency the government was prematurely bundling the elderly into their second childhood. The entailments of 'cocoon' sounded positive as they implied security and safety in a way that was in keeping with the natural world. Drawing on images from nature meant that staying in was really part of a natural process in the growth and development of a species rather than an unnatural imposition by government on personal liberties. However, support is found for a more critical stance towards the metaphor when we realise the verb 'cocoon' was still typically something that people described as necessary for *others* rather than themselves; in the Coronavirus Corpus there only 10 instances when 'cocoon' is preceded by 'we' whereas there are 35 instances of 'cocoon' preceded by 'they' as in:

> To protect their physical health, <u>they</u> must *cocoon* or self-isolate—completely, indefinitely, and some alone.

> Mr. Connolly added: "This could be assistance for an older person with maintaining their ability to stay safe and well in their own home as <u>they</u> *cocoon*, such as the cost of handrails,

> Once a member contracts the virus, can <u>they</u> just *cocoon* together and take the knock?"

There were only 7 instances of the first person singular pronoun 'I' in relation to cocoon and some of these did not reflect compliance:

> When the Government said <u>I</u> should *cocoon* <u>I</u> said <u>I'm</u> not going to sit in the house.

A very common collocation was 'cocoon themselves' as in the following:

> In some ways, this lockdown period enables people to *cocoon* <u>themselves</u> or shield, but now re-engaging with our old lives can sharpen anxiety
>   While visiting grandparents is banned, as the over-70s *cocoon* <u>themselves</u> against the Coronavirus,
>   Unlike in the past, Americans can easily *cocoon* <u>themselves</u> in their preferred media *bubbles*, making a collective response far more difficult.

So in terms of agency, people viewed 'cocooning' as something that *others* were required to do in order to comply with government policy rather than as acts of *personal* volition. As well as from pronoun analysis, this is perhaps why critics of the metaphor used the phrase 'forced to cocoon':

> There is particular concern about the mental health of young people already prone to anxiety and the elderly who have been *forced to cocoon* since the start of the pandemic.[16]

After being *forced to* "*cocoon*" themselves at home since the beginning of lockdown, members of the public classed as extremely vulnerable to Covid-19 are reportedly to be released from self-isolation at the end of July.[17]

The harsh reality of COVID-19 lockdown restrictions for thousands of cancer patients was the feeling of isolation and loneliness, as they were *forced to cocoon* away from family members, receive their cancer diagnoses by phone, and face treatment alone, without support.[18]

In the Coronavirus Corpus there were approximately the same number of instances of 'forced to cocoon' as there were 'asked to cocoon', and the UK press was also sceptical:

People who were *asked to* "*cocoon*" themselves at home for weeks on end could be asked to do so again, Prof Whitty indicated.

But, nevertheless, the press tended to be a mouthpiece for government policy rather than offering more explicit criticism. If older people wished to highlight their own agency, they were more likely to use a different metaphor—that of 'shielding', and this may be why some public policy announcements emphasised this metaphor:

People who were asked to "*cocoon*" themselves at home for weeks on end could be asked to do so again, Prof Whitty indicated.

While the Government relaxed the rules due to concerns over the impact on people's mental health, the chief medical officer revealed that the guidance around *shielding* was now being reviewed as the virus continues to surge.

"The *shielding* patterns are actually being re-looked at," he told a Downing Street press conference. The view about *shielding* is that, in the first wave, *shielding* did many things that were useful but also did many things that were actually actively harmful…".[19]

The metaphor of 'shield' derives from the semantic field of 'war' and this raises the question of what differentiates the two metaphors. 'Cocoon' implies a complete container that encircles the protected individual whereas 'shield' implies only a partial one. Because you have to hold up a shield physically to defend yourself (cocooning is a natural process), 'shielding' implies greater agency on the part of the protected. There were 100 instances of 'I shield' in the Coronavirus Corpus and many of these emphasized agency:

> I *immediately chose to shield*. As a disabled person, I was aware if I contracted the coronavirus, my already limited mobility would deteriorate.
> I've *chosen to shield*—so far as staying at home and only leaving to exercise locally—because I have chronic asthma.
> I tried *to shield* her, but she was in shock. She didn't get any sleep that night, and we were terrified.

With 'shielding' there is the idea of someone taking responsibility for their own actions and this may be why a war-based metaphor rather one deriving from the natural world of butterflies was preferred by people who were emphasizing their own agency. However, both 'cocoon' and 'shield' developed an association with isolation and loneliness; the notion of the cocoon in particular entailed a complete separation that was often viewed as psychologically harmful:

> It is week four of isolation, *cocooning* and whatever else you may want to call it. The cabin fever, anxiety
> Added to this are the effects of isolation and *cocooning*, a completely unnatural way for people to live in 2020
> Consider older and vulnerable people's needs as they re-join communities after weeks of *cocooning* and isolation.
> The presence of this virus in society has further solidified existing issues while further alienating some older people, as we have seen extensive increases in loneliness through the isolation experienced from *cocooning*. We established a loneliness task force to ensure we were putting provisions in place to safeguard older people, presently, and into the future.[20]

There were similar collocations of 'isolation' with 'shielding' especially when viewed from a third person perspective:

> Campaigners are worried the extreme sense of isolation felt by those *shielding*, care home residents and carers during the coronavirus pandemic.

to meet demand for mental health support during the pandemic and is asking the Government about plans on how to safely bring people who are *shielding* out of <u>isolation</u>.

We had admissions from people where they had no history of psychiatric problems, no history of mental health problems, but they were coming in and being admitted because of social <u>isolation</u>, because of *shielding*.

So when 'shielding' was from a first-person perspective it implied agency and volition but a third person point of view undermined this and implied isolation. There was some opposition to the Lockdown on the grounds that freedom was negatively affected by exclusive concern with the needs of minorities: the elderly and those with underlying health conditions. Some thought this was at the expense of the young and the healthy who were unlikely to catch Covid-19 and, if they did, were unlikely to experience serious health effects.

The 'Protective Ring' Metaphor

No group was more vulnerable to Covid-19 than those living in Care Homes—the combination of their age and enforced proximity, both with other elderly people and their care workers, created ripe conditions in which the virus could flourish and it was for this reason that they needed particular protection. When describing the measures that he claimed were achieving this protection, in his Statement of 15th May 2020 the Health Secretary, Matt Hancock, drew on the metaphor 'protective ring':

> Right from the start it's been clear that this horrible virus affects older people most. Right from the start, we've tried to *throw a protective ring* around our care homes. We set out our first advice in February, and as the virus grew, we strengthened it throughout. We've made sure that care homes have the resources they need to control the spread of infection.

He repeated the metaphor twice later in the statement:

From the start, we've worked incredibly hard *to throw that protective ring* around our care homes ... And the point that I think I tried to articulate in my opening comments, is that we've tried to build infection control and the support and *the protective ring* around care homes, right from the start.[21]

'Ring' is a word that carries positive connotations in English, the typical adjectives that describe it are 'nice', 'golden', 'beautiful', 'new' and 'magic'- it is also associated with establishing a life-long commitment to another person in the form of marriage, and I am sure that Matt Hancock would have liked to bring all these associations to mind with this metaphor. Moreover, agency implied by *'throwing* a protective ring' was one that implied a heroic life saver, casting out a lifebuoy ring to a drowning person and he clearly enjoyed depicting a scenario that emphasized the agency of the government in caring for the elderly. It appealed strongly to the moral frame of Care—that is until it was found that he was not being entirely candid with the claim of protection:

The Government did not, as he claims, try to "throw *a protective ring* around care homes". It did the opposite, opening them up to untested patients from hospitals.[22]

Boris Johnson set out his 28-page coronavirus battle plan. It made no mention of *a protective ring* being thrown around care homes but instead instructed care leaders to work together to support early discharge from hospital' with no routine tests for those sent back into care homes. Numerous care home managers have since spoken of how they felt pressurised to take hospital patients.[23]

Right from the start there were critics, and the volume of criticism grew because not only was the Health Secretary being parsimonious with the truth, he actually appeared to be lying:

In evidence that raises further questions about ministers' claims to have "thrown *a protective ring* around care homes", it emerged that agency workers—often employed on zero-hours contracts—unwittingly spread the infection as the pandemic grew, according to the study by Public Health England (PHE).[24]

The 'protective ring' metaphor was one that heightened the agency of the government and in particular the Health Secretary. There are clear transitivity relationships as 'throw' is a transitive verb and one does not 'throw' a lifebuoy ring around oneself, but around someone else, and the viewpoint is from the subject of 'throw'. The function of the 'ring' container, like the 'cocoon' and the 'shield' was to protect, but his opponents claimed that in reality his policies did the opposite: they actually increased the risks of infection with Covid-19 for those many residents of care homes who had come into contact with untested patients from hospitals who were sent out in large numbers to 'protect the NHS'. So, the evidence of Dishonesty mounted: Matt Hancock might have been seeking to evoke a positive moral intuition associated with Care for the vulnerable, but once this had been exposed, and the truth of what was happening on the ground in terms of increased deaths in care homes became evident, the more his lack of candour became apparent the rider of reason was only pretending to be in control. The following humorous and satirical article develops an allegory that undermined the moral intuitions of his 'protective ring' metaphor:

> Indeed, it is kind of best to think of Hancock and his *protective ring* as a very odd, very low-budget Baywatch remake, in which Hancock sprints in very, very, very slow motion towards various care homes and throws his life-saving *protective ring* towards them. Except that there isn't actually *a protective ring* at all, there's just words.
>
> "I have thrown my *protective ring* around you!" shouts the protective ringless Hancock, his eyes alive with the hope that the power of his words will convince them to overlook the demonstrable certainty that absolutely no *protective ring* is there.
>
> In many ways, it's worse. The trouble with *a protective ring* that is retroactively created through words alone, and then subsequently claimed to have been strengthened, is that there is now a fairly large degree of ambiguity over which side of the ring is meant to be the beneficiary of its protection.
>
> Back in the first days of coronavirus, visits to care homes were banned ostensibly to keep the vulnerable safe. Now it is by no means clear whether *a protective ring* is meant to keep coronavirus out or in.[25]

Analysis of the allegory emphasizes the transitivity and agency relations: the purported actions are those of a hero from Baywatch. But the scathing comment that the real purpose of the 'ring' was to protect the speaker rather than the topic of his speech, exposes the moral ineptitude of his policies and his lack of candour in describing them. Trust relies on candour and Honesty and this is central to our moral intuitions during times of pandemic, 'protective ring' was not a candid metaphor.

The semantic prosody of 'protective ring' signals a container that forms a barrier between whatever is within the 'ring' and 'protects' it from whatever dangers are outside and therefore appealed to the moral intuition of Care, however, when challenged or used ironically it introduced the moral intuition of Harm. It is for this reason that we can argue that there was much in common in all the containment metaphors examined so far, 'bubble', 'cocoon', 'shield' and 'protective ring' were all developed in public communication to make separation attractive and necessary by appealing to moral intuitions but they lacked Honesty and candour. They exhorted moral compliance by 'asking' people to cocoon even when they were no longer required to do so by Lockdown laws, so that the physical compulsion of Lockdown was replaced by the moral coercion of particular social groups: people might be able to go outside and do their own shopping, but they clearly did so at their own risk. The government claimed that a 'protective ring' was being thrown around care homes, whereas the opposite was the case as large numbers of patients were discharged into them from hospitals without being tested. The role of metaphor was therefore to engage in a form of moral coercion where legal coercion was no longer deemed necessary. This moral enforcement motivated what was perhaps the most powerful metaphor opposing government policies on Lockdown—a piece of graffiti on a wall in Manchester that stated unequivocally: "The North is not a petri dish'.

The 'Petri Dish' Metaphor

A petri dish is a very specific form of container and the term was used extensively as a metaphor in public discourse relating to the government's response to Covid-19. In biology a petri dish is a form of container used in scientific experimentation for the cultivation and containment of micro-organisms, such as bacteria or fungi. It is a relatively small dish made of glass or plastic and is named after the German bacteriologist Julius Richard Petri. As a metaphor 'petri dish' refers to a contained community that is being studied as if it was a micro-organism in a biological experiment. 'Petri dish' became a widely used metaphor in public discourse during the pandemic when identifying public spaces that encouraged the spread of Coronavirus. On examining UK newspapers for the one-year period from 1st March 2020, there were 500 stories that referred to 'petri dish', in comparison to 199 stories during the exact previous year. On examining the first 100 of these I found only 17 used 'petri dish' literally and the remaining 83 were metaphors. I found a range of public locations referred to as 'petri dishes' and these are shown in Table 7.4; an example of the metaphoric use of 'petri dish' is given in the middle column and the numbers in the right-hand column indicate the number of stories containing the 'petri dish' metaphor in relation to the location indicated in the left-hand column:

Apart from phones, all of these metaphors referred to a location and there was also evidence of the same locations in the Coronavirus Corpus, though with a lower frequency, for example there were none to 'university', only 1 to 'buses', 5 to 'prisons', 8 to 'cruise ships' and 12 to 'schools'. This suggests that the hyperbolic metaphor had a particular appeal in the British media, often because if offered a critical evaluation of government policy by rejecting the moral claims for both Care and Fairness by substituting it with their opposites: Harm and Cheating: it appealed to the elephant of moral intuition by implying that the north was being deceived into being a guinea pig for government control measures and that the government was being Dishonest about this. Typically, articles containing this metaphor were opinion articles in which readers were exhorted to change either their personal behaviour or drew attention to frailties and oversights in government policy.

It is interesting to note that this is a relatively novel metaphor; the earliest use I could find in the British press was in 2003:

Many among a population of more than six billion, a fourfold rise since 1900, live in the rural slums and mega-cities which provide a *Petri dish* for modern plagues.[26]

Table 7.4 A Covid-infected place is a petri dish

Container	Example	N
Buses	Jeremy, who is a father-of-three also stated that "buses are Petri dishes" (*mirror*, 19 March 2020)	212
Universities	Analysis suggests the "petri-dish" of university digs, campuses and halls are the engine driving the latest surge. (*ExpressOnline*, 10 Oct 2020)	184
Schools	Or, rather, children do. Schools are community hubs. They are also viral hubs, *petri dishes* of hot, mucky children sneezing and hugging and wiping snot in unexpected places ... So should we do that? Or, rather than having our children be the *guinea pigs*, should we just wait and see what happens in other countries? (*The Times*, May 21, 2020)	138
Cruise ships	There are fears the ship could become another Diamond Princess, which was described as a *'floating petri dish'* after 10 passengers died and 700 tested positive for COVID-19. (*mirror*, 27 March 2020)	94
Phones	Experts warn phones could be *acting as a petri dish* cultivating the killer microbe and say alcohol wipes should be used twice a day to disinfect the device. (*MailOnline*, 9 June 2020)	70
The North	Politicians in Manchester, Liverpool, Newcastle and Sheffield raged at 'diktats announced without notice' and said ministers were treating the North like a *'petri dish for experimentation'* while the South gets off lightly. (*MailOnline*, 8 Oct 2020)	56
'Chamber' or 'congress'	For members of Congress who are going back-and-forth, they represent sort of *the perfect petri dish* for how you spread a disease (*Guardian*, 29 July 2020)	54
Prisons	Mr Podmore, who is a professor at the University of Durham, said: "In prisons you have *the perfect petri dish* for coronavirus to take hold. (*mirror*, 19 March 2020)	37
Gyms	'Gyms are *like a petri dish*,' said Laurence Gostin, (*Guardian*, 17 April 2020)	28

The next use was not until April 2019 and, following that, February 2020 and it was only in relation to a specific cruise that established the metaphor in British public discourse; this was the cruise ship *Diamond Princess* that became infected with Covid-19. As a result, passengers were isolated on board for nearly a month, bringing attention to the more general threat the virus presented in such confined environments:

Now that we all know what happens to ships when a pandemic hits, how could anyone sign up for what could be a fortnight's imprisonment *on a floating petri dish*? However, the industry has been brought to its knees by coronavirus and will need all the bookings it can get.[27]

The image of the 'floating petri dish' was appealing to journalists with several stories using this phrase, mostly in the second half of February 2020. The infected cruise ship was an especial concern for newspapers such as *The Times* and *The Daily Telegraph* because of their richer, older readerships:

> If there's one place you wouldn't want to be when there's a lethal pandemic sweeping the globe, it is on a cruise ship, or "*floating petri dishes*" as they are sometimes called.[28]

> Yet were any of them regularly referred to as virus incubators, *petri dishes* or germ carriers—standard accusations regularly hurled against cruise ships.[29]

> Coronavirus has hit the cruise industry particularly hard, with ships condemned by critics as "*floating petri dishes*".[30]

It is possible that the *Diamond Princess*, and subsequently other cruise ships, evoked historic memory of so-called plague ships, which were ships infected with plague victims. In June 1348 merchants arriving in Weymouth on a ship voyaging from Gascony brought the plague into the country. The close living quarters of the crew made such ships the primary vectors for disease transmission via the fleas that bit infected rats and then infected crew members. Later ships reserved for carrying plague victims also became known as 'plague ships' as they flew a flag to warn other ships of their hazardous cargo. Ships had long been recognized, as a likely means of transmission of the plague and their monitoring was one of the earliest forms of quarantine:

> Maritime quarantine, introduced in the fourteenth century in an endeavour to prevent the spread of plague … it survived for over 500 years, presumably because, in the absence of knowledge of the ætiology of plague, no method of procedure more likely to be successful could be devised … It is

now recognized that a Port Health Authority must not only take steps to detect plague, human or rodent, afloat or ashore, at the earliest possible moment, but must eliminate conditions in ships and in shore premises which are conducive to the development of an epizoötic … For the detection of plague every ship arriving from a plague-infected port is medically inspected on arrival, but even if there is no evidence of plague-infection on board, such ships are examined daily by a rat-officer until the discharge of cargo is complete.[31]

The historical concept of an infected ship providing a vector for the spread of infectious disease motivated the 'petri dish' metaphor which then broadened to other means of transmission. Initially, it was smart phones that were identified as a 'portable petri dish' with more than half of the stories describing them as such occurring in the first two months of the outbreak. Once a particular image had become established through the cruise ship, it spread rapidly—broadening to other forms of transport including trains:

Sir, Last week my usual service from Stourbridge junction to Birmingham comprised either a six-carriage train, a five-carriage train or a four-carriage train, between 6.30 am and 7 am, and there was plenty of space to stay apart on the platform and on the train. Today there was only one train service with two carriages, and people were packed tightly together. It was the *perfect Petri dish*.[32]

Anyone who has travelled in the UK by train during the rush hour will be familiar with how the overcrowded conditions are insanitary and conducive to the spread of a virus and it is questionable how far passengers paying high costs for their tickets will be prepared to return to them once the pandemic is over. It is certainly the case that the car has proved a relatively secure 'bubble' for enclosed groups even if it has been less so for taxi drivers, a group who have suffered higher rates of infection by Covid-19. If the 'petri dish' metaphor does anything to alert travel companies to public health demands, then its moral intuition can be applauded.

Apart from means of transport 'the petri dish' metaphor also broadened more generally to a range of institutions associated with infection including universities, schools, political debating chambers and prisons:

Infection rates are currently highest among 17–24-year-olds and at least 45 UK universities are tackling COVID-19 outbreaks. However, Professor Susan Michie of University College London, said it was unfair to blame outbreaks at university campuses on students flouting social distancing rules. She said: "With young people arriving from different parts of the country into shared accommodation it's created **a** *human petri dish*.[33]

Other newspapers urged caution on the metaphors that were used to intensify the impact of the virus:

The ABC's Andrew Probyn asks if schools are required to remain open, they are becoming "*human petri dishes*" for the virus. Scott Morrison does not like this question. I think it is important, Andrew, [that] media don't use that alarmist language. I don't think it helps. I would encourage more moderate language on the issues, particularly based on the medical advice you've heard from us day after day on this issue. I would encourage a more measured way of talking about these issues, because I think that can cause unnecessary alarm amongst parents.[34]

Nonetheless, many commentators were still concerned about the re-opening of schools and used metaphor to urge caution:

Or, rather, children do. Schools are community hubs. They are also viral hubs, *petri dishes* of hot, mucky children sneezing and hugging and wiping snot in unexpected places. Here, in the muggy atmosphere of reception, diseases incubate, are rubbed on jumper sleeves, smeared on lunchboxes and then taken home—to spread throughout the catchment area. When school is out, so is the disease. … So should we do that? Or, rather than having our children be the *guinea pigs*, should we just wait and see what happens in other countries?[35]

The phrase 'sneezing and hugging and wiping snot' appeals to another moral intuition—Sanctity and Degradation. The feelings of disgust that are triggered by the idea of 'mucky' children suggest that there is something degrading going on here. The entailment of a metaphor drawn from biological experimentation is that since the biologist is intentionally cultivating a micro-organism in a petri dish, then the authorities are *intentionally* allowing the development of the virus within whatever location is referred to as a 'petri dish'. This is clear in articles where 'petri dish' is used in the context of 'guinea pig' as in the above.

There is therefore an appeal to moral intuition in metaphors of experimentation both as regards the Harm that is caused by deliberately allowing the virus to flourish, the Degrading nature of these experiments and the constraints that they place on Liberty. The petri dish metaphor, like the 'guinea pig' metaphor, reveals human agency—in this case of those who are making the rules about Covid-19—and the moral intuition of the metaphor points to an underlying truth about power relationships. Another intensifier that was used was the phrase 'perfect petri dish':

> infectious disease professor at UC Berkeley, because cruise ships "are a *perfect petri dish* for spreading disease.
>
> Brussels or Strasbourg, the institution is the *perfect petri dish*: Thousands of people gather there from each and every region of Europe,
>
> UK is a crowded country and our capital is a global city—the *perfect petri dish* for a global pandemic.

The last of these proved troublingly prophetic. The morality of the 'petri dish' metaphor shows many of the features that I have identified in other containment metaphors; the perspective here is external to the dish and is cooly observing and commenting on the affected human agent that is contained within the dish. But the additional moral frame that is evoked is the irony of 'perfect', a word that should be applied to Sanctity not Degradation.

An event that was controversially permitted to go ahead in the week leading up to the Lockdown was the Cheltenham races "On social media the mystified called Cheltenham everything from a "*ticking time-bomb*" to a "*human petri dish*". Other forms of hyperbole were used in relation to this event:

> Cheltenham's racing proceedings. Among the many making their way to a *giant Petri dish*, some 20,000 Irish will go and come back with winnings, with stories.

Subsequent infection rates in Cheltenham confirmed the view of many epidemiologists that this was what had become known as a 'superspreader event'. The government was never Honest about the risks involved in allowing the event to run and largely did so for economic reasons. Although the expression 'superspreader' was first used by *The Daily Telegraph* in May 2007, the first use of the full form of this neologism was in relation to a meeting of a biotech company Biogen, as John Carroll noted:

> 'The smartest people in healthcare and drug development—and they were completely oblivious to the biggest thing that was about to shatter their world.' The strategy meeting was one of many examples in the US of a super-spreader event that sees a small gathering generate a huge amount of infections. Other 'superspreader events' included a 40th birthday party in Connecticut that saw around half of the 50 guests become infected.[36]

The concept of the 'superspreader event' soon went viral and the expression has been used in 849 Coronavirus related stories in the UK press since its first use on 18 May 2020. It is interesting that of these 490 stories used the hyphenated form 'super-spreader' whereas 351 used the fully compounded 'superspreader': as the concept became more established so there was a tendency to fully compress the two words into a single word.

In some cases, groups of people defined by their location described themselves as being 'in the petri dish' thereby appealing to the moral frame of Loyalty and Betrayal. This is what occurred following the publicity given to the graffiti daubed on a wall in Piccadilly Gardens in Manchester stating that 'the North is not a petri dish'. This obtained much publicity in the media with 55 stories referring in some way to this metaphor in relation to the north. The strong political message appealed to a moral intuition that government policy was treating the north, and in particular Manchester, as a place of experimentation evoking the same emotion of disgust as we found when 'schools' were described as 'petri dishes'. *The Observer* provided the following summary of the event:

> Somewhere deep in Manchester City Council's storage is a new and unusual piece of modern art. Weighing one tonne, the chunk of concrete

and mangled iron, which previously belonged to a notoriously unpopular partition wall in central Manchester, is expected to make its gallery debut in the new year.

The work will be somewhat familiar to many people, not only in Manchester but across the UK, due to the crudely daubed message in red paint, which reads: *"the north is not a petri dish"*. It is a recreation of the graffiti that made headlines in October when it appeared overnight thanks to the efforts of a mystery vandal.

At the time when Frankie Stocks, the 19-year-old formerly anonymous perpetrator sprayed the message on the wall at Piccadilly Gardens, the pandemic was at a peak in Manchester, and the city's mayor, Andy Burnham, had locked horns with prime minister Boris Johnson over desperately needed help for hospitality businesses in the worst-affected areas. ... This time he was successful and the phrase *"the north is not a petri dish"* became a powerful, resonating symbol for many in the north of England.[37]

The slogan became a rallying cry for the regions to protest against policies believed to favour London and the South-East and so was making a moral comment on the Dishonesty of the government about prioritising its own geographical location at the expense of the north. It viewed the country as a set of regions, each as it were a container of government funding, and argued on the grounds of fairness for the so-called 'levelling up' agenda. This had become the slogan following the Conservative Party's success in the north of England in the 2019 election for raising the economic and social positions of poorer regions, so that they approached those in the rest of the country. Measures of economic position, incidentally, rarely consider differences in the cost of living, in particular accommodation, between different regions. While 'The West' and 'The 'East' may not carry the same political clout, it does not mean they are necessarily any poorer in real terms than 'The North' which also includes a number of quite wealthy areas. Nevertheless, for politicians they had a popular appeal grounded in the moral intuition of Fairness and Cheating and it was for this reason that it was decided to relocate it to Manchester art gallery:

In October last year, graffiti appeared in Manchester Piccadilly Gardens, declaring: *"The north is not a petri dish"*—a critique of the government's treatment of England's upper half during the pandemic. The student responsible, Frankie Stocks, was invited to recreate the slogan after his canvas, a slab of concrete known locally as the Berlin Wall, was demolished before Christmas. The ersatz work is set to go on display in Manchester's Art Gallery later this year.[38]

The 'petri dish' metaphor articulated a moral critique of government policy, unlike 'bubbles' and 'cocoons' that echoed government language, the 'petri dish' metaphor was coined by those who were opposed to the Dishonesty of official policy. This rallying cry appealed to several different moral intuitions, as well as Dishonesty, Harm, Cheating, Betrayal, Subversion, Degradation and, above all, Oppression—and as a result has exerted some influence on government policy.

The 'Bunker' Metaphor

Lockdown measures required people to withdraw to separate spaces where they would be protected from the virus and these were often referred to as 'bunkers'; to emphasise the extent of the withdrawal, this retreat from society was referred to as 'bunkering down'.[39]

> Sydneysiders appeared to follow the premier's request by *bunkering down* at home, with the CBD turning into a ghost town on Saturday night.[40]
>
> I'm at a point where I actually just want to *bunker down* with my family, play my role by (hopefully) not catching or transmitting it, and basically not put my/our heads above the parapet until 1st July and take stock then.[41]
>
> People are no longer so willing to *bunker down* in their little apartments, stepping out in the evenings to applaud courageous nurses.[42]

The verb form of 'bunker' has a metaphoric sense that emphasises the extent that people are separating themselves within a container, as if they were in a military bunker in a time of war. *MailOnline* informed its readers on in a headline:

Chaos in the *Downing Street bunker*: Boris Johnson battles coronavirus from his self-isolation in No11, aides sleep in cabin beds in No 10 while staff struggle to stay in touch as Zoom conferences keep crashing.[43]

And *the Daily Star* told its readers that:

The wartime bunker that could be redeployed in the event of coronavirus breakdown; Demand for secure underground bunker hideouts has soared across the globe and many are relics of our military past.[44]

The idea of a space that was safe from enemy attack was often elaborated in the United States into stories about 'Prepping' and 'luxury bunkers':

'People with money are going to want <u>luxury bunkers</u>. That's what we have here: <u>luxury bunkers</u>' a source said to Bloomberg.[45]

When you're talking about <u>luxury bunkers</u> and survival communities and so on, you're always also talking about capitalist individualism, and the damage it does to the relations between people, the idea of society.[46]

There was often a theme in these stories of contrast between the rich who had access to a 'bunker' and the rest of society who did not. *The Independent* ran a story entitled: "GOING TO GROUND; Unprecedented as it is, some believe the current crisis is a warm-up for what comes next. Bradley Garrett gets to know the bunker builders preparing for the end of the world."[47] Unlike 'cocoon' and 'bubble' which were containment metaphors developed by governments to motivate the people to protect, and the 'petri dish' metaphor that resisted these socio-medical policies, the 'bunker' metaphor was one that emphasised individual responses to the pandemic and rejected any broader appeal to moral intuitions other than survival and care for one's immediate kin.

The 'bunker' became a metonym for disasters in general and this showed in the expression 'bunker mentality' that indicates this extension beyond any actual military situation to a state of mind associated with separation and detachment:

If the hoped for and much needed V-shaped recovery is to transpire then we must banish the *bunker mentality* and venture out from behind our four walls.[48]

As argued in relation to the 'war' and 'fire' frames in Chaps. 2 and 3, the pandemic evoked a **general disaster frame** that brought on ideas of a zombie apocalypse as previously discussed in Chap. 4; *The Times* explained the appeal of this sort of thinking:

There are now 40 people living in the community where each bunker costs $35,000. "They have all got their American flags. Some of them have put fences around theirs, so it looks like a cul-de-sac in a suburban area," Garrett says. "Some of the underlined bunkers are really elaborate and beautiful. They've got stainless appliances and wind turbines and solar panels, and others are a little more spartan. It's kind of like a ship. What you've stocked, and the time it allows you, defines the space: can you make it through three weeks, three months or a year?" He argues that the survivalist instinct runs deep and that gated communities are another version of the "*bunker mentality*" going into effect. "This is a distinctly human attribute to prepare for the future. Most animals don't live with this sense of dread and anxiety," he says.

The author goes onto to highlight the psychological advantages of withdrawal to a 'bunker':

For the preppers it is a vindication of all their fears. "People are retreating all over the country right now to their bunkers. A lot of them started going four or five days ago, some of them are just leaving now because they had to wrap up their affairs. I'm getting a barrage of emails from people saying, 'We're going.' It's so weird because I've been talking to them for years about how bad does it have to get before you pack up your house and go to the bunker? And this is it. We are in the time when all the doomsday preppers are pulling the ripcord. The first night in my bunker, I had the best night's sleep of my life".[49]

The pandemic provided the right conditions for Preppers' fears of the collapse of society and vindicated their prior behaviours, and costs, in the construction and provision of their bunkers as places of safety for their tribe. The author is probably right in emphasising the motivating force of fear and anxiety in determining human behaviour, but the idea of acting *before* a disaster hits also motivates arguments for a pre-emptive strike against a perceived opponent when they are perceived to be weaker. One of the main arguments against nuclear weapons has always been because of the inherent immorality of inflicting a disaster on others on the assumption that they might inflict a disaster on you.

One of the problems with such dystopic beliefs is that they do not encourage the type of social engagement that is likely to prevent societies from the sort of collapse on which they are presupposed; bunker builders tend, like conspiracy theorists in general, to believe that they have some *privileged knowledge* that enables them to *know* the real dangers *before* everyone else; although proactive, they also reflect **individualistic, atavistic and fear-driven thought** species survival is enhanced by moral intuitions based on large scale co-operation rather than narrow individualism.

The 'Pod' and 'Pocket' Metaphors

The word 'pod' developed during the Coronavirus period to refer to any form of enclosure that was erected to control spread of the virus:

> NHS England has refused to say how much it paid for the 15 isolation pods it bought but the Norwegian-built plastic-covered stretchers normally cost around £35,000 each.

> A gym has reopened with individual pods to help people maintain social distancing while working out in a bid to prevent the spread of coronavirus.

> Care homes are using glass visitor pods during the second lockdown so residents can still see their family. ... Northfield, which has 63 beds, bought the glass pods using local government infection prevention and control (IPC) funds.

> "Despite the fact contestants have to stand in a studio with no clothes on, they actually reveal themselves from behind disinfected glass pods which can be wiped down afterwards."[50]

Since these are all material structures of some sort, 'pod' can be treated as polysemous as these senses are extensions of the earlier sense of 'elongated seed pod' but as metaphors when they refer to non-material entities such as:

> So I organized *a learning pod* at our house with other quarantined families. We have seven kids and two teachers. And it's absolutely amazing![51]

> But you really shouldn't have sex with people outside of *your quarantine pod*. Public health expert and former FDA official Dr. Charlene Brown said sex should still be off the table with strangers and roommates, as there's a high chance of being infected with COVID-19 even if you're hooking up with someone you live with.[52]

In such cases 'pod' is an alternative to other metaphoric containers such as 'social bubble' as it describes a group of people who are intentionally restricting contact with others. 'Pod' suggests intimacy and cosiness, it is because a seed pod is small that its seeds are packed in close together. It also has a greater solidity than 'bubble' because of the more established extended meaning of some form of barrier that creates a *complete* separation from whatever surrounds it. As with 'bubble', 'pod' implies a three-dimensional entity that offers 360-degree protection; unlike a shield, that is a more two-dimensional structure, 'pod' conveys a higher level of security from infection. However, typically a 'pod' is transparent as it is usually constructed of glass or plastic: people can be observed in their 'pods' from a point of view that is typically outside the pod, evidence for this is that the collocation 'your pod' is much more frequent than 'our' or 'my' pod.

Another containment metaphor that was used quite extensively was 'pockets' as for example in the phrase 'pockets of infection' which occurred over 100 times in the Coronavirus Corpus:

> Scientists and ministers are concerned that vaccination hesitancy, particularly in deprived areas, could create "*pockets of infection*" which continue to fuel transmission and slow down the efforts to ease lockdown.

South Africa has been lauded for its aggressive effort to root out *pockets of infection* with screening and testing, as well as its big economic relief package.

By acting quickly against *pockets of infection*, the virus would, in time, be suppressed to the point of virtual elimination without needing to close down the entire economy.

The phrase referred to the identification of social or geographical areas in which the virus was active with a view to some form of government-initiated intervention. The concept of 'pockets of infection' implied these areas were relatively small and therefore it was possible to take effective action within them. However, the phrase was only used in the plural implying that, although not large, there were a number of these infected areas and therefore a social response was necessary. Along with 'pod' the notion that something is known and being acted upon was intended to convey a sense of knowledge about the virus and therefore had the purpose of reassuring the public about the public health response.

An interesting feature of the phrase 'pockets of' is that it was often followed by a negative entity; these included 'poverty', 'poor', 'violence' and 'corrupt' and these negative evaluations carried over to human entities that were described as 'pockets of' and that were only negative depending on the perspective of the reporter, such as 'protesters':

The march comes after *pockets* of protesters in central London clashed with police during a demonstration on Wednesday.

There are fears that *pockets of* unvaccinated people in difficult-to-reach areas will not only result in further illness and deaths, but also provide a pool for dangerous new variants to develop.

The agency attributed the outbreaks to travelers who got measles abroad and *pockets of* unvaccinated people.

Most importantly, he didn't seem the least concerned to oversee that the money be actually spent on tackling COVID-19 and not end up in the *pockets of* corrupt politicians and terrorist groups.

There is no particular reason why the pattern 'pockets of x' should imply a social evil of some sort and so the effect here is 'semantic prosody' whereby the associations of typically negative senses of 'pockets of' carry over to other contexts so that the listener or reader is primed for thinking that whatever entity is in the object position of 'pocket of' is probably a negative social phenomenon. It is by such means that moral intuitions are expressed linguistically.

Notes

1. Chmara, T. (2015). "Do minors have first Amendment Rights in Schools?" *Knowledge Quest*, 44(1): 8–13.
2. https://www.auckland.ac.nz/en/news/2020/06/03/pm-metaphorical-view-covid-19.html. Accessed 26 June 2021.
3. https://www.odt.co.nz/star-news/star-national/here-are-rules-alert-level-3-and-2-lockdown. Accessed 26 June 2021.
4. https://www.expressandstar.com/news/health/coronavirus-covid19/2021/01/01/nhs-in-eye-of-the-storm-and-under-enormous-pressure-treating-covid-19-patients/. Accessed 26 June 2021.
5. *US Fed News.* 2 June 2020.
6. *Express Online* 10 Sept 2020.
7. *The Guardian,* 21 December 2020.
8. *telegraph.co.uk,* 19 December 2020.
9. *mirror.co.uk,* 24 November 2020.
10. BNC = British National Corpus.
11. https://www.etymonline.com/word/bubble.
12. Robert Fisk, *The Independent* 24 March 2020.
13. Robert Fisk, *The Independent* 19 June 2020.
14. Jenni Russell, *The Times,* 25 June 2020.
15. June 28, 2020.
16. https://www.irishtimes.com/news/health/ireland-post-pandemic-facing-a-tsunami-of-mental-health-problems-1.4273850. Accessed 26 June 2021.
17. telegraph.co.uk, 18 June 2020.
18. https://www.theparliamentmagazine.eu/news/article/covid19s-cancer-legacy.
19. *telegraph.co.uk,* 31 December 2020.
20. https://psychcentral.com/news/2020/07/25/pandemic-fuels-feelings-of-loneliness-anxiety-in-people-over-70/158212.html. Accessed 26 June 2021.

21. https://www.rev.com/blog/transcripts/united-kingdom-coronavirus-briefing-transcript-may-15-with-matt-hancock. Accessed 26 June 2021.
22. *The People*, 12 May 2020.
23. *MAIL ON SUNDAY*, 17 May 2020.
24. *The Guardian*, 18 May 2020.
25. *The Independent*, 19 May 2020.
26. *The Observer*, 27 April 2003.
27. *The Times*, 3 July 2020.
28. *The Daily Telegraph*, 3 April 2020.
29. *telegraph.co.uk*, 21 April 2020.
30. *The Times*, 25 March 2020.
31. White C.F. (1935) Plague: Modern Preventive Measures in Ships and Ports. *Proceedings of the Royal Society of Medicine* 28(5): 591–602.
32. *The Times*, 24 March 2020.
33. *Express Online*, 2 October 2020.
34. *The Guardian*, 23 March 2020.
35. *The Times*, 21 May 2020.
36. *MailOnline*, 13 April 2020.
37. *The Observer*, 20 December 2020.
38. *The Guardian*, 5 February 2021.
39. There were 173 uses in UK press stories and more than 100 occurrences in the Coronavirus Corpus.
40. *MailOnline*, 19 December 2020.
41. https://community.eurogamer.net/thread/339171?start=6180. Accessed 26 June 2021.
42. https://www.washingtonpost.com/world/europe/covid-europe-second-wave-lockdowns/2020/10/28/e0f2d9b2-1863-11eb-8bda-814ca56e138b_story.html. Accessed 26 June 2021.
43. *MailOnline*, 28 March 2020.
44. *The Daily Star*, 10 April 2020.
45. *MailOnline*, 1 April 2020.
46. https://thespinoff.co.nz/books/23-07-2020/the-man-who-looked-the-apocalypse-in-the-face-and-laughed/. Accessed 26 June 2021.
47. *The Independent*, 10 June 2020.
48. *Express Online*, 22 August 2020.
49. *The Times*, 26 March 2020.
50. *Daily Star Online*, 2 July 2020.
51. *MailOnline*, 2 December 2020.
52. https://www.dailydot.com/irl/coronavirus-sex-bdsm/. Accessed 26 June 2021.

8

Metonyms of the Pandemic

Introduction

When we think of the aftermath of war, we may gain a measure of the destruction by imagining a film taken from a small aeroplane flying over the ruins. Everywhere piles of rubble, the empty shards of multi-storey buildings with their floors collapsed and the staring black holes of their windows like empty eye sockets. Astonishingly, there are also a few fine domes and spires that are still untouched, their untarnished beauty all the more remarkable by contrast with the surrounding destruction. But what is the immediate aftermath of Covid-19? Just empty streets, wide circular roads normally teeming with traffic are now empty, cats strolling around. Boulevards that should be packed with pedestrians going about their daily business are now vacant except for a solitary cyclist: the last survivor of an apocalypse. The effect of a mass pandemic is not a destruction of the infrastructure of the city but of its inhabitants, as if some dirty bomb had finally gone off and all that was left was a drone capturing the event for an audience on a remote planet or in an underground bunker. Somehow the photographer does not look for metaphors, but for the single image that captures the entirety: the beautiful dome that rises above the chaos

J. Charteris-Black, *Metaphors of Coronavirus*,
https://doi.org/10.1007/978-3-030-85106-4_8

of rubble, a cat not even needing to look to left or right so confident is she of the absence of danger. These images are *metonyms* not metaphors, because the pile of rubble or the shells of buildings are from the same semantic field as that which they signify: the devastating effects of a disaster. A metonymy 'involves only one conceptual domain, in that the mapping or connection between two things is within the same domain'.[1] While ultimately conceptual, they can be expressed by images, in which case they are visual metonyms[2,3] or by words. In both cases they are one shot takes that encapsulate the whole story.

What might be the metonyms, or visual metonyms, of the global pandemic of 2020? I accidentally left my diary for that year in a Motorway Services café and did not bother to replace it, but an empty diary might be considered a metonym: a redundant object in a vacant world. A discarded disposable mask blowing down the street. A lonely girl staring out of a window. An old lady talking on a phone to a younger woman standing outside in the street also holding a phone. A bright red and orange shuttered-up amusement arcade. A man wearing a hazmat suit pushing a trolley stretcher along a hospital corridor. A large city cinema with empty film hoardings with a billboard promising: "We'll be back again soon". A man cycling on his exercise bike alone in a kitchen. Laundry hanging on a clothes dryer. A long black hearse driving slowly up a hill. A woman talking to the tiny face of a child on a screen. These are metonyms that answer the question: "is this what it has all come to?"

Because these images are selected for our attention within the context of the pandemic, they reduce *multiple* thoughts and emotions to a *single* object, or event. The mask signifies an attempt to avoid catching an airborne disease—it is a CAUSE-EFFECT metonym so that 'Are you properly masked?' means "Are you fully protected"? Metonyms draw on a much larger context than that which they actually depict by simplifying it to a single object. The mask and the hazmat suit—whether shown in words or images—are metonyms for the Covid-19 pandemic because they bring to mind a salient, but everyday, experience of the pandemic. Film and photography are the natural language of the pandemic because although an, much of our experience was on our own, we continued to bear witness by taking images. Even when we were not able to converse and we were left alone with our thoughts, emotions and reflections we could still share understanding with images. While the casually discarded mask blowing along the road may evoke a reflection on who its owner might have been and what happened to them, it is also just a discarded mask: metonymy reduces the multiple and complex to the singular and simple.

Taking Gibb's definition further: metonymy is "a cognitive process in which one conceptual entity, the vehicle, provides mental access to another conceptual entity, the target, within the same domain…".[4] But given the all-encompassing nature of the pandemic surely *everything* had the potential to be interpreted metonymically? Given this definition and the qualification, in this chapter I try to answer the question: what can metonymy tell us about the pandemic? By identifying metonyms from the British press, I consider the extent to which the following conceptual entities provided mental access to the experience of the pandemic: the mask, the hazmat suit, the hearse and the rainbow. 'Mask' was too frequent a word to identify the number of Coronavirus stories, so Table 8.1 only shows the frequency of the remaining 3 metonyms in different British press reports:

The sample shown in Table 8.1 could equally have included other conceptual entities that were metonyms for Covid-19: a bottle of hand sanitiser, a syringe or a vial containing the vaccine, protective gloves, a full-face visor, or wipes, but with metonymy selection is both necessary and subjective.

Metonymy in the Naming of Disease

Metonymy is commonly practiced in the naming of diseases by eponyms; diseases can be named after the person or medical expert who first identified the disease, for example 'Alzheimer's' after a German psychiatrist Alöis Alzheimer, or by using the name of the first known case of the disease, for example 'Lou Gehrig's disease' after the American basketball player of that name; these follow the metonym PERSON'S NAME (EXPERT OR VICTIM) FOR DISEASE. Another metonym is to name the disease by its symptom as for example 'respiratory disease', or 'smallpox' following the metonym SYMPTOM FOR DISEASE. A further practice is to name a disease after an occupation with which it is

Table 8.1 Frequency of 'pandemic' metonyms in the British Press (2020–2021)

	Feb	March	April	May	June	July	Aug	Sept	Oct	Nov	Dec	Jan	Feb
Hazmat suit	37	117	49	42	26	33	8	30	15	6	20	9	4
Hearse	0	11	59	45	19	9	11	6	17	22	4	37	15
Rainbow	10	139	465	384	192	143	82	94	117	90	129	112	107

associated; so, for example we have 'tennis elbow' and 'mad hatter's disease'; there is also 'Legionnaires Disease' named after people who went to a convention of the American Legion in Philadelphia in 1976; these, broadly, follow the conceptual metonym OCCUPATION FOR DISEASE.

Another way of naming a disease is by using toponyms where the proper name for a place refers to a disease that originated in a particular location following the metonym PLACE OF ORIGIN FOR DISEASE. Although it is **not** the practice recommended by The World Health Authority (WHO), toponyms are often employed in the naming of disease: Spanish flu, the British, South African, or Indian variants, or even the names of regions as in the 'Kent variant'. The WHO prefers the greater objectivity of numbers such as 'B.1.617.2' rather than 'Indian variant'. This preference was partly a reaction against terms such as 'China Virus' that Donald Trump had coined and repeatedly used while he was President. The phrase 'China Virus' co-occurred with 'Trump' in 783 different British press reports. However, the first use I could find was in a headline from *The New York Times*: "China Virus Kills 22 and Sickens Thousands", (3 May 2008) and the first use in the UK was also in a headline: "Wuhan pneumonia: Mystery China virus is from same family as Sars, scientists say; 'A novel coronavirus could not be ruled out,' says the WHO".[5] It seems that the sensationalism of headline writers does not always comply with a preference for non-prejudicial disease names.

Sometimes the use of place names can have the effect of stimulating metaphoric thought, because if a place is represented as the origin of a disease the conceptual metonym PLACE OF ORIGIN FOR DISEASE can extend into a further metonym PLACE FOR INFECTED PEOPLE. Through generalization, based on part-whole relationship the infected people in a location can be taken to represent the *whole population in that location*; there is then a conceptual metaphor: THE OUT-GROUP IS DISEASED and, by inference, THE IN-GROUP IS HEALTHY. Thinking of 'self' and 'other' in terms of the *cause* of infection and in terms of place or location can therefore contribute to negative representations of people from elsewhere, immigrants, foreigners or just people from another city or region when they are defined as carriers of disease. Implicating a geographic location as the source of a disease with the metonymy PLACE FOR INFECTED PEOPLE risks implying that *all* people from this place will carry with them that disease. Although travel really does increase the likelihood of microbe transmission, hence the practice of quarantine, it is unlikely that this is always the case. It risks creating the fallacy that it is *only* the outsider who can 'carry' the disease, whereas, in reality, it is infected natives who are *unaware that they have the disease* who present a greater danger. The WHO noted:

> While they have their advantages, these scientific names can be difficult to say and recall, and are prone to misreporting. As a result, people often resort to calling variants by the places where they are detected, which is stigmatizing and discriminatory.

As a result, in May 2021 they proposed the following alternatives which are summarised in Table 8.2:

Proposing alternative names does not guarantee that they will be adopted, either by scientists, the media or by the general public. Although the removal of metonyms in the naming of diseases is motivated by considerations of Care and Harm and seeks to establish a fairer and more honest terminology for diseases, there is some research to indicate that there is no strong effect of metonymic disease naming such as 'China virus' or 'Wuhan virus' on xenophobia:

> To conclude, this paper provided the first empirical test of the psychological effects of infectious disease naming. The key takeaway is that naming did not impact levels of sinophobia or anxiety, risk perceptions, and beliefs about the pandemic. Therefore, returning to the goal of "First Doing No Harm" (Fukuda et al. 2015), governments, media outlets, and international bodies can be more assured that their choice of name for an infectious

Table 8.2 New names for Covid variants (WHO)

Location of origin of variant	WHO name	Scientific name
Kent	Alpha	B.1.1.7
South African	Beta	B.1.351
Brazil	Gamma	P.1
India	Delta	B.1.617.2

disease is unlikely to lead to harmful xenophobia or negative psychological impacts, and thus they might be best served to focus their limited resources elsewhere.[6]

The research is based on two separate studies across three countries (the US, Canada and India) and, although its findings seem rather counterintuitive, it warns against making automatic assumptions that place metonyms are necessarily xenophobic, since there is a long history of indicating provenance, for example of food products, by toponyms.

The Mask

Prior to Covid-19 mask-wearing as a social practice was largely restricted to the wealthier parts of Asia, one imagined young tourists from Japan going about in their skinny jeans, their intelligent eyes peering through black-rimmed glasses over a white or floral mask. Wearing masks, at least outdoors, had been a practice in Japan since the Spanish flu: educational posters featured slogans such as "reckless are those who don't wear masks." But it had much earlier origins:

> Covering the mouth with paper or the sacred sakaki (Japanese cleyera) leaves to prevent one's "unclean" breath from defiling religious rituals and festivals has been common from ancient times, Hirai says, and is a custom still observed at Yasaka Shrine in Kyoto and the Otori Grand Shrine in Osaka, among others. During the Edo Period (1603–1868), the practice seems to have penetrated a significant portion of the population.[7]

In Zoroastrian religious practice the magi, or priests, would wear a mouth cover, (known as a *padan*) to prevent their breath sullying the Sacred Fire. In the west, prior to Covid-19, mask wearing was, wrongly, believed to be for the wearer's *own* protection rather than from a desire to avoid contaminating *others*. Growing awareness of the potential for reciprocal protection offered by masks was part of a new global awareness in public hygiene practice. It was advised that masks would not protect their wearer nearly as much as it would protect those in their vicinity and for this reason mask-wearing became legally enforceable in indoor public spaces in many parts of the world.

The topics discussed by the press included whether or not mask-wearing should be voluntary or mandatory, and, if the latter, which groups (if any) should be exempted; for example, should children wear them? Should they be worn everywhere or just in specific locations such as public transport and should they be doubled up? Then there were the masks themselves: how could you get hold of them? Should you make them yourself? What was their efficacy and how was this affected by the fabric, fit, design, number of layers etc. whether, or not, they were reusable and, if so, how many times? Could they be washed? Should they be ironed? Were they a style item, or purely a public health requirement? What could be done about the effect of glasses misting up? One topic that was avoided was that since mask-wearing was traditionally a practice associated with female sexual modesty, especially in Muslim cultures, did the mask make someone more, or less, alluring? There is an argument that masks enhance appeal by bringing more attention to the eyes, contrary to their intended effect in Muslim cultures. Concealing the lips and mouth the mask still offers a hint of their contours. Journalists addressed mask-wearing more in terms of practical, and possibly life-saving, concerns with more enthusiasm than they had scientific evidence to support their arguments. They rarely considered cultural or aesthetic considerations. During the pandemic the mask shifted from being a metonym for religious affiliation, or for female modesty to one for protection of others.

For several years, I have been a collector of masks, I have wooden masks from Java representing the characters of the Ramayana, colourful masks from Sri Lanka and Ivory Coast, unpainted masks carved by the indigenous people of Malaysia, masks made from clay and feathers from New Guinea, others made of metal or plaster and some that I have made myself from stones and shells collected from British beaches. I am attracted by the combination of textures, colours and the weight of the different materials and how this interacts with the emotional expressivity of the human face. I like the ideas behind their use in ritual, whether to dispel illness, or bring about a change of state in the wearer or the viewer.

But these masks are *not* the ones that you think of in relation to the Covid-19 pandemic, which brings to mind a surgical mask covering the mouth and nose rather than the whole face. So, the concept of MASK is now quite different from before the pandemic: it now has a medical sense, rather than one related to cultural meaning or ritual practice. The domain of public health has come to exclude cultural domains, so that 'mask' takes on the metonymic sense of 'protection' and pushes out its richer metaphoric senses. While the metaphoric meaning of masks is something that reveals inner truths by concealing identity, the metonymic meaning of mask is simply a screen for self-protection and the protection of others. Yet, according to a book entitled *State of Fear* the official response to Covid-19 was worse than the disease itself; in this argument masks were a means for enforcing social conformity: "The behavioural psychologists love masks. … They promote collectivism, the feeling that we are all 'in it together'". The author goes on to argue that:

> Behavioural scientists pushed for masks because they create a 'signal', when in fact not a single Randomised controlled trial can demonstrate the value of mask-wearing outside of clinical settings. … they are a visible indicator that there is danger present all around, in the air we breathe and in the people we meet. Masked faces prime you to think of danger. We become walking billboards for disease and danger. They keep fear in our faces. Literally, they also distinguish the compliant from the rebels….[8]

The author argues that the British government coercively manipulated the population to compliant behaviour by making fear the central message of a propaganda campaign. The book continues: "The unintended consequences of the masks is that they keep the fear alive and modify our behaviour…"[9] It would seem to me that this was not unintended at all—surely the whole purpose of wearing a mask is to raise awareness of risk and so modify behaviour? What her analysis fails to consider is that the British government was not alone in developing a policy for influencing social behaviour during a pandemic. Governments across the world were obliged to respond to Covid-19 and in many cases employed much more rigorous social controls that included enforcement of complete quarantine. In France they needed a document to go outside and in Spain over 1000 people were arrested for violating social distancing regulations in March 2020 and there were fines of 60,000 euros for repeated violation of quarantine. In Brazil where Bolsonaro adopted a highly libertarian approach there were over half a million deaths. This was an international health emergency to which governments everywhere were responding to high infection levels and death rates. Given the UK's high death rate, there was a case for much stricter quarantine policies and higher levels of enforcement of infection control measures such as mask-wearing. Of course, there were inevitably marginal psychological impacts, but surely the psychological impact of losing a relative to Covid-19, or experiencing 'Long-Covid' was also not negligible? Populist messages that rejected lockdown confirmed the biases of the audience they were written for—and those putting them forward, like proponents of miracle cures, often did so as much for financial gain as moral perspective. My argument is that a lack of honesty in public communication, combined with the moral turpitude of some government officials that allowed them to break the rules they had themselves created, added grist to the mill of such anti-lockdown morality.

In terms of moral frames, the metonymic meaning of 'mask' is related to the moral intuition of Care and Harm based on the metonym of CAUSE FOR EFFECT in which wearing a mask stands for protecting and being protected. This differs from the metaphoric senses of masks in cultural practice where they can signify Loyalty or Betrayal, Sanctity or Degradation. Audiences in Hindu-related mask-wearing performances know the character, and even soul, of the wearer from the evidence of the mask. While most authorities agreed that masks offered some form of protection, a few experts deemed them harmful, and their views were circulated on social media:

The claims, often made in widely shared social media posts, sound alarming. Face masks increase the risk of catching Covid-19; they suppress the immune system; wear one long enough and they'll push up your blood pressure, starve the body of oxygen and allow carbon dioxide to build to toxic levels.[10]

In reality, though, there were other more metaphoric or symbolic reasons for wearing, or refusing to wear, masks beyond practical health considerations. Some wore masks as badges of loyalty and support for more interventionist responses by government to the pandemic, while other 'anti-maskers', as illustrated above, refused to wear them, treating them as symbols of oppression. For anti-maskers the right not to wear a mask was an expression of freedom, something as fundamentally human as the right to breath. With this metaphoric and ideological meaning of mask-wearing, both 'maskers' and 'anti-maskers' displayed their tribal affiliations based on opposing stances deriving from different interpretations of their moral intuitions regarding Loyalty and Liberty. *Not wearing* a mask was a statement of affiliation with a libertarian position that held that constraint on individual human behaviour by government was an oppressive power grab, this is the line taken in *State of Fear*. This anti-mask viewpoint reflected the traditional liberal notion of negative freedom which argued that the State should not have the right to infringe the rights of the individual to be unconstrained.[11] Not wearing the mask was an ideological way of asserting the liberty of the individual based on the concept FREEDOM IS NOT WEARING A MASK. By contrast, wearing a mask was a statement of affiliation to an ideology that asserted the rights of society over those of the individual and implied that social freedom could only come from behaviour based on the concept FREEDOM IS WEARING A MASK.

Drawing on Isiah Berlin's interpretation of the distinction between negative and positive liberty, the action of mask-wearing therefore expressed positive liberty because the survival of individuals depended on the state imposing restrictions on *not* wearing a mask, even if they appeared authoritarian. This was presumably the position of traditionally liberal newspapers like *The Guardian* that took a strongly interventionist approach that limited individual freedoms: wearing a mask restricted a small amount of the individual's freedom in exchange for a much greater freedom from illness for the group. This could be seen as paradoxical when measured by negative liberty and the paradox is only removed when it is interpreted as an expression of positive liberty.

Another moral intuition that mask-wearing, or not mask-wearing, appealed to was Authority and Subversion: if you were forced to wear a mask by a source of authority that was enforced by security guards, then *not* wearing one was a means of *subverting* this authority. The metonymic meaning of the CAUSE FOR EFFECT metonym is that, like wearing a seatbelt, or a cycling helmet, wearing a mask results in protection. This appealed to the moral frame of Care and Harm, but anti-maskers placed a more metaphoric meaning on mask wearing based on OPPRESSION IS MASK-WEARING. *MailOnline* summarises this viewpoint:

> The most outlandish have spread from America, where there is growing opposition to mask- wearing despite a terrifying surge in coronavirus cases. They are linked mainly to far-Right Christian groups who refuse to wear them and have staged demonstrations about their 'right to breathe … Images from the US on social media show people carrying exemption cards from the 'Freedom To Breathe Agency'.

This ideological standpoint was reflected in the coinage of the name 'anti-masker', that was linked with 'Covid denier'. Pro-maskers were the liberal-left who were motivated by the CAUSE FOR EFFECT metonym and the moral intuitions about Fairness and Cheating, but they were prepared to appeal to other intuitions such as Loyalty by wearing masks depicting a national flag. Closer analysis of how the anti-mask movement took off in July 2020 in some parts of the world shows that, while stories occur in the British press, they are typically reporting events in Australia or the United States, and their ideological basis is summarised as follows:

> The Gallup poll also revealed that US mask-wearers and anti-maskers are largely divided along party lines, with 75% of Democrats but fewer than half of Republicans saying they had worn a mask in public. … In April, Donald Trump undermined the CDC's recommendation that the public wear masks, saying he was 'choosing not to do it'. The idea that wearing a mask signals submissive weakness or a forfeiture of individual freedoms has also gained currency with some anti-maskers.
>
> The first protest to kick off was the Stand for Freedom Ohio rally which saw hundreds of attendees collect to stand against mask mandates. According to ABC 6, the anti-mask protest was advertised as an open-carry event where 'security' would be provided by 'militia, military veterans,

bikers and patriot groups'. The group also spoke out against coronavirus shutdowns and in favor of the police.

Armed men and women in camouflage surrounded the protest, many others wearing American flag clothing. Several of the protesters were seen waving Trump 2020 signs as they brandished firearms. 'I will not wear someone else's fear' signs read, as others called for schools to be reopened. 'Let out people go. We don't need masks. We don't need out businesses shut down,' one protester told ABC. 'We are free.'[12]

Moral intuitions of Loyalty expressed themselves in a series of demonstrations where the right to freedom was articulated by an ideological rejection of the mask as a symbol of fear, rather than as a metonym for protection, and the meaning of the mask became metaphoric rather than metonymic.

The following anecdote illustrates the ideology of mask-wearing: one cold day in February 2021 I had just gone into my local supermarket and my glasses steamed up, as often happens with a sharp temperature change. In order to navigate the store (following the maze of arrows glued to the floor) and to see the produce I had lowered the mask so that it only covered my mouth rather than my nose as well; a young man approached and told me that I was not wearing my mask properly: in his eyes I was Cheating by wearing a mask but not in a way that offered proper protection: for him I might even be a covert anti-masker! For him FREEDOM IS WEARING A MASK PROPERLY. I wondered whether his concern was for my welfare as an individual, for the welfare of others, or as a display of Loyalty to the pro-mask ideology? I think the latter. A similar sentiment was expressed by a Harry Potter star called Jason Isaacs:

> I am less annoyed by the people who don't wear masks, who should be in the stocks or prison, but the people who don't wear it over their nose. Or the people who pull it down to have a chat and then pull it back up, they should be hanging in the streets![13]

I would suggest that in these cases mask-wearing had gone beyond being a metonym for protection based on Care/ Harm but had become a metaphor for a whole set of left-wing moral and political values.[14] I describe this as an ideological metaphor because here mask-wearing is pointing less towards considerations of CAUSE FOR EFFECT disease transmission and more towards to a general political stance.[15]

By October, another peak of 'anti-mask' reporting, the issue had extended to the online battle between warring ideologies:

> Membership to Facebook groups promoting anti-mask arguments has risen by nearly 2000 per cent since August, new analysis has revealed.
>
> One group with more than 3000 members urges members to invite all their Facebook contacts to join in order to promote the message. "Absolutely no pro-mask posts will be approved and anyone commenting with pro-mask bulls**t will be removed from the group," it states.
>
> Facebook said it is actively cracking down on the spread of misinformation relating to coronavirus and removes claims that directly contradict advice given by WHO that would lead to imminent physical harm.
>
> "We remove any anti-mask claims that could contribute to risk of imminent physical harm, and we reduce the distribution of false claims that have been fact checked and show warning labels with more context," a spokesperson told *The Independent*.[16]

Evidently the mask had taken on a fully ideological meaning that went far beyond its metonymic one.

An example of this switch from metonym to metaphor can be found in the debate on mask wearing on Twitter where masks are referred to by libertarian anti-maskers and Covid deniers, as 'muzzles'. The word 'muzzles' co-occurs with either 'anti-mask' or 'anti-masker' in 34 British news reports during the period that were related to an ideological stance on freedom of speech:

> Some people oppose the new mask rules not just because they think they're ineffective, but because they see them as an unfair intrusion on personal liberty. They call the move "dystopian" and often refer to the masks as "muzzles".[17]

> The new rules are contentious, with some people finding masks uncomfortable and some libertarians complaining they are being "muzzled" by the state.[18]

The use of quotation marks here is an indicator of metaphor, as a muzzle would normally be worn by an animal and typically a dog. Isabel Oakshotte posted a tweet on 14 July 2020:

> Muzzles should be voluntary, not mandatory. Another sinister encroachment of the state! @michalegove was right—keep the law out of it; and let people exercise their common sense.

It was 'liked' 4100 times, received 4600 comments and was retweeted 1700 times. The moral intuition to which she was appealing was that of Liberty and was based on the conceptual metaphors OPPRESSION IS MASK-WEARING and FREEDOM IS NOT WEARING A MASK. There were many who shared the sentiment that mask wearing infringed their liberty, but the use of 'muzzle' introduces an explicit metaphor frame into the mask debate: the muzzle is worn (usually) by a fierce dog to constrain its mouth and has connotations of restriction, oppression and domination relationships: someone puts a muzzle on someone, or something else whom they wish to control. So, the 'muzzle' metaphor introduces the concept of an external source of authority that infringes on personal liberty. The 'muzzle' metaphor, along with the sheep icon, was extensively adopted by anti-maskers in the social media debate on mask-wearing. Evidently, the mask as a CAUSE FOR EFFECT metonym was contested and both libertarian and anti-libertarian ideologies gave metaphoric meanings to mask-wearing that went beyond the medical function of the mask to its role as an ideological badge.

The Hazmat Suit

The hazmat suit is a very different type of metonym from the mask: whereas the mask was an ideologically disputed symbol that took on metaphoric as well as metonymic senses this was not the case with the hazmat suit: the hazmat suit became a metonym for complete protection. As we have seen, prior to the pandemic the mask symbolised a range of meanings from ideological commitment to the traditions of Islam to cultural practices involving spirit transfer, largely because it covered *the face:* the primary source of identity. By contrast, the hazmat suit was a garment that required complex design so that it covered *the whole body* and therefore was necessarily limited to the specific domain of bodily protection. While previous infections had aroused awareness of the need for protective equipment, such as the hazmat suit, for medical staff, it was not until the Coronavirus pandemic that it became a recognisable metonym for the specific illness of Covid-19. The brightly coloured complete wrap around garment with gloves, boots, fitted mask and voluminous presence soon came to symbolize the techno-scientific response to the crisis—just as the orange jumpsuit worn by prisoners at Guantanamo Bay had previously become the metonym for the terrorism crisis of the post-2003 period. The two garments had very different referential frameworks: the hazmat suit brought status and authority to the wearer whereas the orange jumpsuit removed their status and authority. The protective function of the hazmat suit reflects in the fact that the largest number of reports referring to it occurred at the onset of the global pandemic in March 2020 (see Table 8.1) and that it generally reduced in its newsworthiness after that month. In this respect we can consider the hazmat suit as a metonym for the peak rates of covid-19 infection: it symbolized the epicentre of the crisis in the United Kingdom.

Inevitably protection creates a barrier between the patient and the medical personnel whose role it is to care for them; the contact of human flesh is now no longer feasible and even eye contact is indirect, but the expense in making a hazmat suit allows the wearer to accrue the prestige of an expert. Like its progenitor, the beaked helmet and long gown worn by plague doctors, the hazmat suit served as a metonym for the pandemic: it would only be worn for this condition in circumstances of medical emergency. As with its precursor the beaked helmet, the very sight of the hazmat suit was sufficient to evoke conflicting emotions. The fear of diagnosis with a terminal illness might conflict with the desire for treatment that could sustain life, as in the following:

> The patient realises they are no longer just a person, but a vector of disease. A hazmat suit looming over you—well, it's not something you ever want to see. But it is better than the alternative: a lonely room, with no medical intervention at all. Because, although the person in a hazmat suit may seem

far away, or even uncaring, they are doing the most humane thing imaginable: putting themselves in harm's way, to save a stranger's life.

The same journalist uses the metaphor of 'armour' for the garment (my italics):

> The hazmat suit creates a barrier between humanity and nature. Nature is conceived as hostile, full of threat. ..."The virus is a revenge of nature," Lynteris says. "It decimates humanity, and then nature flourishes." The hazmat suit represents humanity's resistance to this existential crisis. *Like a knight going into battle in a jangling suit of armour*, the epidemiologist dons the hazmat suit to *wage war on nature*.[19]

The journalist relishes activating the war frame, which, as we have seen, was viewed more positively in the early stages of the pandemic than later on. The metaphor adds a touch of heroism: just as only aristocratic knights could afford metal armour for their jousts, so the hazmat suit became an elite garment that conferred status and authority. This may be why the sight of the suit in everyday contexts would create a sense of the surreal that demanded attention as indicated in the following report:

> A shopper was spotted browsing the aisles of a Tesco Extra store wearing a full hazmat suit and gas mask as the nation continues to be gripped by coronavirus panic. The man appeared to be stocking up on meat, filling his trolley with trays of mince and some kind of joint. Fellow shopper Ethan Mees says he was shocked when he spotted the man in the Yeovil store in Somerset.
>
> Mr. Mees, who was shopping with his father Jeremy at the time, says he saw the person at the shop on Queensway Place at around 11 am today ... He said: "Everyone in the shop was looking at him." I was shocked and so were a lot of people and the staff. I was with my dad just shopping and spotted the man dressed in an all-in-one suit, rubber shoe covers, gloves and a mask.[20]

The shopper is not framed as a heroic warrior but as someone who may be mentally unstable and who needs careful observation. A similar frame for mental instability is activated by the following:

The suspected Covid-infected passenger dragged off a plane by Hazmat-suited medics showed 'no symptoms' and received a text only seconds before take-off 'saying he was positive', a fellow flyer has claimed.[21]

A PASSENGER at Dublin Airport stunned travellers by wearing a Covid-proof hazmat suit on her flight home for Christmas.[22]

Just as wearing a mask had previously been something that bandits did to conceal their identity, so the metonym of the hazmat suit could carry with it metaphoric senses implying instability and abnormality when worn by non-professionals in unexpected settings. Unlike the ubiquitous mask that could be seen everywhere, it was a situation-specific metonym.

The hazmat suit usually featured either in stories about generic classes of worker, cleaners, hospital staff etc., who were wearing it for protection in a Covid-infected environment and so was a metonym for the rate of infection and hence the severity of the crisis in that location. In other cases, celebrities were reported because they were wearing one: there were 44 reports on Naomi Campbell wearing a hazmat suit and there were other stories in which the England cricketer Jofra Archer and Russia's President Putin wore one. In some cases, the metonym of the hazmat suit stood alongside other metonyms such as the mass grave and the morgue that all form part of a morbidity frame for the pandemic:

Drone footage shows inmates in hazmat suit digging graves on NYC's Hart Island suggesting that coronavirus victims could already be being temporarily buried there, as morgues across the city continue to overflow and the death toll ticks up.[23]

The connection between metonyms was used by the Indonesian government in its public communication:

The authorities have already resorted to displaying empty coffins at busy intersections in the capital, Jakarta, as a reminder of the risks of the highly contagious virus. The coffins, next to a mannequin in a protective hazmat suit, have been painted with the words "Covid-19 victim" in red, to drive home the message for people to take necessary precautions.

The coffins, that I examine in the next section, were presumably insufficient in themselves to activate a morbidity frame that was specific to Covid-19.

In terms of metonymy the hazmat suit proved to be generally resistant to metaphor and tended to retain its metonymic sense of complete bodily protection, although it was a covert marker of status and prestige because of its cost. As it was a rather surreal and foreign garment its alien-like quality gave it a symbolic meaning: the movement of the body in a hazmat suit is necessarily slower, constrained and rather like a zombie. As a *Daily Mirror* reporter commented:

> It took me 194 redials to get my hairdressers appointment, and then I hated every weird, alien second of it. The necessary safety precautions—me in a mask and enormous plastic poncho, stylist in basically a Hazmat suit—only reiterated that I was taking a risk.[24]

Similarly, a reporter for the *Independent* referred to the hazmat suit as symbolising strangeness:

> Unless you intend to live in a hermetically-sealed unit or wear a hazmat suit 24/7, life goes on. … Coronavirus feels unreal. It is as if we're living through an even lower-budget 28 Days Later or Invasion of the Body Snatchers. An alien force enters our lives and we're powerless to stop it.[25]

The very strangeness of the pandemic—it's evocation of a zombie apocalypse—was perhaps best symbolized by the hazmat suit.

The Hearse

The word 'hearse' originates from a combination of metonymy with metaphor. It is derived from the Latin word *hirpex* meaning 'harrow'. Originally, a wooden or metal framework was needed over the coffin to hold it in place and to support the pall or covering. To perform this function effectively it was designed with numerous spikes; these extended downwards to secure the coffin or bier and covering but could also extend upwards to serve as candle holders. Because these spikes resembled the teeth of a harrow, it became known as a hearse. This is an appearance-based metaphor because the harrow-like teeth were the salient visual aspect of the 'hearse'. Later on, the word was applied, not only to the framework above the coffin, but to any receptacle on which the coffin was placed: this was a metonym because the framework and the coffin were literally adjacent to each other, or contiguous in experience. The idea of 'harrow' disappeared for most and the metaphor was therefore lost. Then, from about 1650, 'hearse' came to denote the vehicle on which the coffin was transported to the place of burial. This was a further metonym because the coffin was literally placed on or into the vehicle.

In terms of cognitive frames, the hearse is the vehicle that transports the coffin to the place of burial and is part of a scenario involving the death of a human being, whose body must then be managed in such a way as to respect its dignity, the emotions of those who knew the loved one and the broader sense of acknowledgement required by social decorum. The hearse as a vehicle draws on the conceptual metaphors DEATH IS A DEPARTURE and DEATH IS GOING TO A FINAL DESTINATION frame (Lakoff & Turner 1989). In classical mythology death was a journey across the River Styx, a journey filled with immortal significance, and in any society the passing of a dead body brings complex emotions reminding us of all those who have died, and indeed of our own future death. It is common to stand respectfully, in silence, and sometimes to cross the heart, or to take-off a hat or even to cast flowers upon the passing vehicle. The hearse gives cognitive access to the whole experience of death as part of a ceremonial acknowledgement of the material transition of the deceased human body to its final resting place where we hope that DEATH IS SLEEP.

From my top floor apartment on a busy arterial road of Bristol I could glance at many vehicles moving up and down the hill and I noticed how many more hearses were moving around the city during the first Lockdown, not an hour would go past without a hearse going by: time and space merged in this visual reminder of death. I would typically think first of whether it was on the way to collecting a body or, having already done so, was moving on to the next stage of the journey. Then I would consider who the deceased had been, who their family was and what emotions they might be feeling. It is the tradition for a hearse to drive slowly and in a dignified way with the driver carrying a suitably serious demeanour. But it was difficult to see the vehicle without bringing to mind the scenario of events that comprised this final journey to a final destination.

In the British press, not a single report contained 'hearse' in February 2020, this had soon changed to over 100 reports in the months of April and May (see Table 8.1). Unsurprisingly, the curve on a graph for the frequency of 'hearse' in the British press mirrored the curve of the UK death rate. In very few of these was the hearse the main topic of the article, although this could occur:

> In Rotherham, South Yorkshire, a heart-warming video showed the moment a group of strangers rushed out to help a hearse up a hill after it got stuck in the snow.
> Michelle Mulcahy, 40, who watched from her living room, said it "restored my faith in humanity". The hearse was headed to the nearby crematorium before sliding to a halt.[26]

Others referred to the hearse simply as a metonym for the experience of death within a close-knit community:

> "I know five people who've died, people who've been around since I was little. They had years ahead of them. We can't attend the funerals because they're restricted, so we all tend to go out in the street when a hearse goes past just so the family knows they are in our thoughts." Dorothy Lewis has been running her tiny grocery store in Tylorstown for 53 years.[27]

Here the hearse is a passing reminder of the loss of a member of the community and the bereavement of a family; it leads Dorothy to reflect on the number of others she has known who have recently died. Often the death of a known person served as a metonym for the social management of death. In an article about a funeral home director in a small-town in Louisiana, *The Guardian* reported on the changing nature of the business during Covid-19:

> Because he was raised in a funeral home, Charlet knows how to prepare for the worst. He was taught at a young age to fill up the gas tank on the hearse

before the local high school prom, in case there were deaths resulting from drunk-driving accidents.

But even Charlet wasn't prepared for the Covid-19 pandemic. "The first couple of months, it was really scary because there wasn't a lot of guidance on what we were supposed to do," he said. A short supply of body bags meant some bodies had to be wrapped in sheets....

Charlet has a printout of an essay called Always Go to the Funeral by Deirdre Sullivan in a folder of clippings he wants read at his funeral. "Humans kind of need that ritual of saying goodbye," he said. "You have to acknowledge someone's death."[28]

Here the hearse is taken as a starting point for cognitive access to the whole concept of running a funeral business and the huge increase for their services that the pandemic caused: it stands for the social acknowledgment of death and for this reason the hearse, rather more than the coffin, serves as a metonym for the Covid-19 pandemic.

The Rainbow

By April 2020 in the United Kingdom the rainbow had become the people's symbol of support for the efforts made by National Health Service workers and also one of a united-front against Covid-19. You could barely walk along a road anywhere in the country without seeing a window displaying the colourful arc of the rainbow. Typically, it was drawn and coloured by children and could be made from any medium from paint, to paper flowers, to multiple cut out hearts or stars. Rainbow enthusiasts sometimes painted a huge one on the external walls of their house. These rainbows located on the private space of the home, looked outwards, rather than inwards, so that the home became a sort of window to the world beyond the home. *MailOnline* online summarised the positive psychological motivations behind the symbol:

And even those who cannot offer any material goods have been spreading cheer by sending supportive messages, in particular to NHS workers on the front line of the coronavirus fightback. Thousands of households across the

UK are also placing children's drawings of rainbows in windows 'to brighten the community during the coronavirus pandemic'.[29]

The message of reassurance could be reinforced verbally as explained the *telegraph*:

> Children around the world are painting rainbows to hang in their windows to raise the spirits of passers-by. The trend has become popular in the UK since schools closed. PA reports that in Oldham, Vicky Corbley's children posted a rainbow in her kitchen window, with the messages "don't worry" and "we'll get through," with messages thanking delivery drivers and postal workers.[30]

It is worth noting that the powerful image of the rainbow did not originate from government communication experts, according to the *telegraph* it had a much humbler originator: a young woman on furlough, who, having seen one in Italy, created a Facebook group initiative:

> The rainbow is the undeniable symbol of 2020: a message of hope, something to spot on a daily walk, and a way of showing our key workers that we are thinking about them. And it was all started by Crystal, a 32-year-old mum who was furloughed from her job in a nursery when she came up with the idea back in March.
>
> Crystal had seen a picture of the rainbow as a symbol of hope in Italy. She decided to make one for her window with her four-year old year old daughter, Ariana, and suggested others follow suit on local Facebook groups. Within days, thousands of families were posting pictures of their creations. 'Some people covered their whole houses in chalk. It was amazing,' she says.[31]

The social media-initiated image of the rainbow became a symbol of response to the pandemic at a local level and communicated a sense of social alignment with community values; Table 8.1 shows that the number of news reports on the topic of Coronavirus that included the word 'rainbow' peaked in April but there were still over 100 reports per month through May, June and July and only dropped below that figure in August and September, to rise again in the autumn with the Second Wave. The rainbow had become a quiet message that—rather than opposition towards an out-group—appealed to a sense of solidarity among the people—a sort of universal in-group. Most people would have little difficulty in interpreting the meaning of the rainbow as a symbol of hope, as the BBC explained:

> In Christian culture, a rainbow promises better times to come—the Abrahamic god sent one to Noah after the great flood as a sign that people could go forth and multiply without fear of another calamitous drowning. Rainbows are frequently represented in Western art and culture, as a sign of hope and promise of better times to come.[32]

Some might think the rainbow is a metaphor because the sense of hope is more abstract than the experiential phenomenon of light refraction; however, I view the rainbow as a visual metonym because the image gives conceptual access to something that is part of the same domain as the meteorological event: if when you see a rainbow, you automatically experience a feeling of hope and point it out to whoever is with you at the time, it is surely partly because it makes you feel optimistic? Because the interpretation of a rainbow as hope is so deeply rooted in cultural knowledge, they are both part of the same conceptual domain and therefore the rainbow image is a visual metonym.

By 'cultural knowledge' I am not claiming that most people are necessarily aware of the biblical sign sent by the Christian God to Noah (though many would be) but I *am* suggesting that the optimistic state of mind we know as hope occupies the same conceptual space as 'rainbow'. Evidence for this might be if you asked 10 people to draw a symbol for hope, the majority would draw a rainbow. If this is the case, then the rainbow accesses through the visual mode the same concept as is expressed by the word 'hope'. Further evidence is that if you look at images of the rainbow depicted in people's windows only a few of them actually say 'hope'- they might refer to the NHS, or say 'thank you', 'stay safe', 'be confident', 'we are all in this together' but it is taken for granted that the rainbow means 'hope'- so it is redundant to write 'hope' as part of the sign. If this is the case, then we might think of the rainbow as a visual metonym, one embedded deeply in the culture, and probably widespread around many cultures although, as we saw above, it derives from the Bible:

[12] And God said, "This is the sign of the covenant I am making between me and you and every living creature with you, a covenant for all generations to come: [13] I have set my rainbow in the clouds, and it will be the sign of the covenant between me and the earth. [14] Whenever I bring clouds over the earth and the rainbow appears in the clouds, [15] I will remember my covenant between me and you and all living creatures of every kind. Never again will the waters become a flood to destroy all life. [16] Whenever the rainbow appears in the clouds, I will see it and remember the everlasting covenant between God and all living creatures of every kind on the earth."

[17] So God said to Noah, "This is the sign of the covenant I have established between me and all life on the earth."[33]

As Covid-19 reaped its grim harvest across the planet, it is worth reflecting whether or not at some level, people felt a need to *remind* God of his covenant: perhaps believers felt that God had forgotten them. I overheard a woman saying in Pawson's greengrocer's in Bishopston, Bristol "x has died and y has died, and you know I don't believe in God anymore, I just don't believe". So, the visual metonym of the rainbow—unlike the hearse, the mask or the hazmat suit—was one whose purpose was to offer reassurance and to dispel fear of the present and doubt about the future.

However, not everyone was enamored of the rainbow, in her account of the government's strategy for dealing with Covid-19, Laura Dodson argues that behavioural science and nudge theory was employed as part of a general strategy to frighten and manipulate public opinion. The author of *State of Fear*, expresses her suspicion of the rainbow and other manifestations of government propaganda such as 'Clap for Carers': "I bristled at the rainbows in people's windows. It felt like a clap for Boris rather than a clap for the NHS. I think governments used it as a shield".[34] However, it seems that she searched among her interviews for anything that would confirm her own bias against Lockdown to produce an account that would appeal to an audience of those who were opposed to Lockdown or thought that Covid-19 was not really so much to worry about—especially given its damaging psychological effect. She suggests that putting rainbows in the window was unconsciously motivated by more magical beliefs about the power of talismen to ward off disease.

Other symbols such as the green man, or a lucky horseshoe, or in Arabic culture, wearing a symbolic eye to protect against the evil eye, have contributed to other rituals of protection that derive from pre-scientific thinking.[35]

Given the ubiquitously positive emotions that are generally associated with the rainbow and its metonymic association with hope, it is not surprising that this was not the first campaign of its type to employ it as a symbol. Since 1978 the rainbow had been a symbol of gay pride. It was inspired by the artist Gilbert Baker who designed the first rainbow flag to signify gay pride. Similarly, following the abolition of apartheid in South Africa, a new multi-ethnic identity was expressed by the term 'rainbow nation' which originated in Nelson Mandela's inaugural speech:

> We have triumphed in the effort to implant hope in the breasts of the millions of our people. We enter into a covenant that we shall build the society in which all South Africans, both black and white, will be able to walk tall, without any fear in their hearts, assured of their inalienable right to human dignity—*a rainbow nation* at peace with itself and the world.[36]

Here the reference to 'hope' and the archaic word 'covenant' alludes to the Bible but the use of 'rainbow' as a premodifier of 'nation' turns the phrase into a metaphor, as there is the novel idea of a national recognition and embrace of the reality of a nation comprised of people of different ethnicities and hence diverse colours. Another use of the word was by the environmental organisation Greenpeace that named its flagship 'Rainbow Warrior'; unfortunately this didn't prevent two agents of the French intelligence services from planting explosives on the ship and sinking it. In spite of their initial denial, this was later proven by investigative journalism to have been an act of state terrorism. It was approved by the French government of the time under President Mitterrand. A photographer, Fernando Pereira was trapped and drowned in the sinking ship. Unfortunately, the rainbow aspirations of the ship came up against a state warrior.

In some cases, experts employed the metonym in relation to the arrival of a vaccine for Covid-19, Monica Gandhi, an infectious disease specialist at UC San Francisco said:

With the "*rainbow of hope* that vaccines are coming", health officials should also signal that an end is in sight, "and let Californians know exactly what they're planning to do to support workers and businesses in the meantime", she said. "We need to understand and acknowledge people's lived experiences in devising policies."[37]

Here the phrase is employed to emphasise the psychological benefits accruing from expectation of a vaccine. In a few cases the folkloric belief that there is a crock of gold hidden at the end of rainbow was employed with the sense of unrealistic expectation of a vaccine as in the following:

> Chancellor Rishi Sunak is among Cabinet ministers said to be warning of the harm more restrictions could have on the fragile recovery from the first lockdown. Tory former minister Lord Vaizey warned the country will have to live with the virus and it is time to "level with the public. You cannot wait for the vaccine *at the end of a rainbow*," he told Times Radio.[38]

He employs the image as part of an argument against a second Lockdown and argues that because we didn't yet have a vaccine it was unrealistic to plan around the possibility of one being developed. Interpretation of 'end of the rainbow' is arrived at through recognising the cultural allusion to the Irish folkloric belief that leprechauns were distrustful of humans and so buried a crock of gold at the end of a rainbow so that only they could find it. In context, it refers to the expectation that something is simply too good to be true and is therefore unreal.

The popularity of the rainbow metonym surprised many: why should a relatively simple symbol prove to be so inspiring, and what did it inspire? It is quite possible that the sense of social cohesion to which the rainbow contributed, appealed partly because it was a *new* symbol for British national identity. Although it had been used in South Africa, it was not the same old slogan from Second World War instructing us to 'Keep Calm and Carry on' and it was not a flag either. It expressed a more vibrant and contemporary image for Britain, one that overcame other possible divisions. In doing this it may well have contributed to a culture of solidarity that was crucial in encouraging uptake of the vaccinations once they became available. But why should a rainbow take on the meaning of social cohesion? An answer is given when we examine the difference between an *actual* rainbow and the sort of rainbow that is depicted in the stylised representations of the NHS rainbow. An actual rainbow is comprised of seven colours that *gradually blend* into each other: we cannot see the boundaries between each separate band of colour. But this is not the case in the painted NHS rainbows, or most other stylised versions of the visual metonym, as each band of colour is usually quite *separate* so that they typically show seven separate arcs that are attached to each other but produce an overall 'rainbow' effect. I think an interpretation of this is that completely diverse entities—people from different social, ethnic, or religious backgrounds—each represented by a separate band of colour, can combine to produce a single unified arc that is more beautiful (or at least more colourful) than any one of the individual arcs of which it is comprised—a metaphor for society. The rainbow therefore expresses the idea *E Pluribus unum* (out of many come one) which provided much needed psychological reassurance at a time of pandemic crisis.

Notes

1. Gibbs, R.W. (1994) *The Poetics of Mind: Figurative Thought, Language, and Understanding.* Cambridge: Cambridge University Press, p. 322.
2. Forceville, C. (2009). Metonymy in visual and audiovisual discourse. In: Eija Ventola and Arsenio Jésus Moya Guijarro (eds), *The World Told and the World Shown: Issues in Multisemiotics.* Basingstoke/New York: Palgrave Macmillan, pp. 56–74.
3. Feng. W.D. (2017) Metonymy and visual representation: towards a social semiotic framework of visual metonymy. *Visual Communication,* vol. 16(4): 441–466.
4. Kövecses, Z. (2010). *Metaphor: A practical Introduction.* New York: Oxford University Press. p. 173.
5. *The Independent,* 9 January 2020.
6. Masters-Waage, T. C., Jha, N. & Reb, J. (2020). COVID-19, Coronavirus, Wuhan Virus, or China Virus? Understanding How to "Do No Harm" When Naming an Infectious Disease. *Frontiers in Psychology* Vol. 11.
7. *The Japan Times,* 4 July 2020.

8. Dodsworth, L. (2021) *A State of Fear: How the UK government weaponised fear during the Covid-19 pandemic*. London: Pinter & Martin, pp. 113–114.
9. Dodsworth, L. (2021) *A State of Fear: How the UK government weaponised fear during the Covid-19 pandemic*. London: Pinter & Martin, p. 237.
10. *MailOnline*, 11 July 2020.
11. https://plato.stanford.edu/entries/liberty-positive-negative/#ParPosLib. Accessed 26 June 2021.
12. *MailOnline*, 18 July 2020.
13. *MailOnline*, 29 September 2020.
14. The term 'woke' is often used, often ironically, to refer to this ideology. For a discussion of 'woke' see https://metro.co.uk/2020/03/27/word-woke-became-tool-silence-people-colour-12426214/. Accessed 26 June 2021.
15. For a discussion of 'ideological metaphor' see Charteris-Black J. (2017b) Competition Metaphors & Ideology: Life as a Race. In R. Wodak and B. Forchtner (eds.) *The Routledge Handbook of Language and Politics*. Routledge: London & New York. Pp. 202–217.
16. *The Independent*, 2 October 2020.
17. *thesun.co.uk*, 17 July 2020.
18. *MailOnline*, 25 July 2020.
19. *The Guardian*, 26 March 2020.
20. *mirror.co.uk*, 13 March 2020.
21. *MailOnline*, 28 August 2020.
22. *Daily Mirror*, 19 December 2020.
23. *MailOnline*, 7 April 2020.
24. *Daily Mirror*, 22 July 2020.
25. *The Independent*, 5 March 2020.
26. *Express Online*, 16 January 2021.
27. *mirror.co.uk*, 30 January 2021.
28. The Guardian, 26 December 2020.
29. *MailOnline*, 20 March 2020.
30. *telegraph.co.uk*, 25 March 2020.
31. *telegraph.co.uk*, 27 December 2020.
32. https://www.bbc.com/culture/article/20200409-rainbows-as-signs-of-thank-you-hope-and-solidarity. Accessed 26 June 2021.
33. https://www.biblegateway.com/passage/?search=Genesis%209&version=NIV. Accessed 26 June 2021.

34. Dodsworth (2021), p. 94.
35. Dodsworth (2021), p. 180
36. https://www.africa.upenn.edu/Articles_Gen/Inaugural_Speech_17984.html. Accessed 26 June 2021.
37. *The Guardian*, 8 December 2020.
38. *Express Online*, 20 September 2020.

9

Magic, Miracle Cures and Metaphoric Thought in the Anti-Vaccine Movement

Introduction

In this chapter I consider how metaphor was used to refer to misinformation strategies regarding Covid-19 and discuss the metaphors that commented on both advocates of bogus remedies and those who exposed them as unscientific. In the first section I discuss expressions such as 'silver' or 'magic' 'bullet' and other magic-related metaphors to demonstrate how they were employed to evaluate Covid-19 remedies, sometimes by dismissing them as childish. In the second section I explore the phrase 'miracle cures' and consider the metaphors that were used to describe their proponents, I also illustrate the range of 'miracle cures' that were on offer. In the third and final section I discuss how the anti-vaccine movement took its origin from human-animal metaphoric thought, but I also illustrate how metaphoric thinking underlies pro-vaccine rhetoric. In each section I suggest that metaphor was crucial in framing the debate and in articulating deeply held moral arguments drawing on religious and humanist philosophical positions that were based on moral intuitions concerning Honesty and Dishonesty.

© The Author(s), under exclusive license to Springer Nature Switzerland AG 2021
J. Charteris-Black, *Metaphors of Coronavirus*,
https://doi.org/10.1007/978-3-030-85106-4_9

Since the eighteenth century western scientific approaches have gradually replaced the use of magic for the treatment of illness and disease in modern societies. Evidence-based research conducts random control studies on a sample of the population to identify efficacious medicines and vaccines. At no time was this more the case than in the search for a vaccine for Covid-19 once the scale of the pandemic became evident. Multibillion dollar contracts were signed with the large research laboratories such as Pfizer and Astra Zeneca for the development of a safe vaccine. The scramble was on as governments mobilised to find a vaccine, while other resources were directed towards testing and imposing quarantine measures. Since there was a gap of unknown duration between the outbreak of Covid-19 and the time when a vaccine might become available the emphasis was on obtaining protective equipment for healthcare staff and testing. In the meantime, the virus was spreading. Since there was no immediate remedy to relieve global anxiety, it was hardly surprising that various magical cures were soon on offer: this was the perfect opportunity for snake oil salesmen, quack doctors and purveyors of traditional remedies. Some political leaders gave their endorsements to dubious and unreliable medicines that were at best placebos and at worst fatal, while spiritual leaders advocated prayer and attention to the afterlife. As Keith Thomas pointed out more than 50 years ago in *Religion and the Decline of Magic*:

> If magic is to be defined as the employment of ineffective techniques that allay anxiety when effective ones are not available, then we must recognise that no society will ever be free of it.[1]

Thomas identifies a basic contrast between religion and magic: religion provides overall explanations of man's purpose while magic is directed towards specific, temporary problems, and Covid-19 presented people everywhere with very specific, though sometimes longer term, problems. In the absence of a remedy for this existential threat from medical science, perhaps some other solution might be found? Populist leaders around the world such as Donald Trump, Jair Bolsonaro in Brazil and Thabo Mbeki in South Africa felt under pressure to come up with a solution since they had never been shy about diagnosing societal 'diseases' and offering their own 'remedies'. They responded to this weight of expectation: based on early findings from a study in France,

Donald Trump, soon followed by Jair Bolsonaro, advocated hydroxy-chloroquine as a miracle cure and Thabo Mbeki, argued for nutritional remedies such as beetroot juice, lemon peel and raw garlic. In India some politicians from the Hindu nationalist BJP party advocated the drinking of cow urine and in Nigeria, a traditional ruler of the kingdom of Ife claimed a combination of plants including onions, African pepper and neem tree could offer protection. It was natural that in societies where people deferred to their leaders in existential matters, these same leaders should provide routines of reassurance based on appealing to the elephant of intuition rather than the rider of reason. However, many were Dishonest in that the remedies they proposed lacked the validity of medical science. Magic is fundamentally a form of deception and a particular metaphor relevant to Thomas's claim was the expression 'no magic bullet' with which scientists and politicians sought to lower public expectations of a vaccine for Covid-19. Of course, they recognised the emotional pressure behind the desire for an easy and straightforward solution to the crisis, but they also sought to divert subsequent blame by going on the record as rejecting a 'magic' or 'silver' 'bullet' solution—whether in the form of a vaccine or some other as yet undiscovered cure. Magic was in the air and drew on deeply held intuitions rather than on reason.

Silver/Magic Bullets and Deceptively Simple Solutions

The metaphorical sense of 'silver bullet' traces its origin to myths and legends claiming that evil forces—werewolfs and witches—were susceptible to a *silver* bullet rather than an ordinary one. The silver bullet gives its possessor superior powers over opponents and was adopted by the American fictional hero the Lone Ranger as his calling card. It is because there are legendary claims for the 'silver bullet' that the phrase is nearly always used in its negative form, 'no silver bullet' implying that it is unrealistic to think that there would be a simple solution:

> "There is *no silver bullet* when it comes to tackling coronavirus," said Baroness Dido Harding, executive chair of the test and trace service.[2]

Covid vaccine approved for Australia rollout but PM warns jabs '*not a silver bullet*'.[3]

The metaphor makes its moral claim by appealing to the speaker's honesty in exposing deception. Those responsible for public health wanted to buy time for research into vaccines by avoiding promises of a 'silver bullet'. The phrase occurred in 753 reports in the British press in the year from 1st March 2020; of these 'not a silver bullet' occurs in 198 reports and 'no silver bullet' occurs in 185 news reports such as these:

The Director General of the World Health Organisation said he hopes there will be a number of effective vaccines to help prevent people from infection but he said 'there's *no silver bullet* and there might never be'.[4]

A vaccination is *no silver bullet* for Covid-19, writes Prof Raj Bhopal CBE, Emeritus Professor of public health at the University of Edinburgh.[5]

Imran Ahmad Khan Wakefield told MPs: "There is *no silver bullet*, and without one, although difficult, we must learn to live with the virus. The continued peaks and troughs are unsustainable and offer false hope."[6]

Sometimes it was policy areas that were not instant or simple solutions:

Mr Raab insisted more airport testing was *not a 'silver bullet'*. 'Let's just be clear about this when we think about airports—there is *no silver bullet* in airports,' he told BBC One's Andrew Marr Show.[7]

There is *no silver bullet* with this virus and efficient, accurate testing in the community is the only solution for the next five years at least.[8]

Of course, while denying that there is a 'silver bullet' is a way of lowering expectations for a specific solution to a specific problem, it does not undermine hope. When vaccines and medicines were not available, research into them was motivated by the hope that in the future they might be. In this respect 'no silver bullet' was not a rejection of the possibility of ever finding a remedy, but rather an exhortation for patience and allowing time for its development. In this regard the appeal to the 'no silver bullet' metaphor is part of a rhetoric of lowering expectation for a 'quick fix' solution—rather than ruling out the possibility of a future remedy. This is an important distinction because for resources to be directed into medical science it is vital that there is at least the *possibility* or *hope* of a remedy—otherwise why bother? We need to recall, then, Keith Thomas's words, that magic could still re-emerge in relation to specific problems for which science had no solution: when the rider of reason loses control the elephant of intuition takes over. 'Silver bullet' as a warrant therefore argues for caution in accepting uncritically any inadequate remedies on offer while the experts are developing vaccines. When combined with 'bullet' a similar cognitive blend occurs with 'magic' as with 'silver': both select one aspect of the schema that we have for a 'bullet' which includes the idea that it can protect from danger and therefore offers a solution to a problem. This complex blend when applied to Covid-19 is represented in Fig. 9.1:

In the first input space we have 'silver' or 'magic' and its schema includes *what it is*: a precious metal in the case of silver (its ontological sense)—and *what it purports to do* in the case of magic: it can be used to change something (its teleological sense); in the second input space we have 'bullet' and its schema includes both the *ontological* sense of *what it is*: a metal projectile and the *teleological* sense of *what it can do*: harm or protect. The senses that transfer from these schemata in the blended space are governed by the ontological and teleological knowledge located in the generic space that is concerned with finding solutions to problems. When interpreting the phrases 'silver bullet' or 'magic bullet', the mind looks for qualities that the adjective and the noun share such as selective *ontological* knowledge of their properties (value) and the *teleological* knowledge of what they *can do*. The reason for the partial suppression of the ontological meaning of 'silver' is that we know it would be wasteful to make a projectile from a precious metal, so the sense of silver as a purchasing medium is suppressed. It is the abstract knowledge from the generic space that drives the selection in the blend and creates the meaning of 'silver/ magic bullet' as an effective means of overcoming problems. In the case of Covid-19 the emergent space comprises the vaccines that medical science are developing. But, of course, there are, or more likely are not, 'silver' or 'magic' bullets for *any* social problem. 'Magic' also evokes a frame for childish games that are inappropriate in a mature adult world and the metaphor 'no magic bullet' is based on an association between magic and deception and so represents speakers who propose deceptively simple solutions as Dishonest because they rely on intuition rather than on reason.

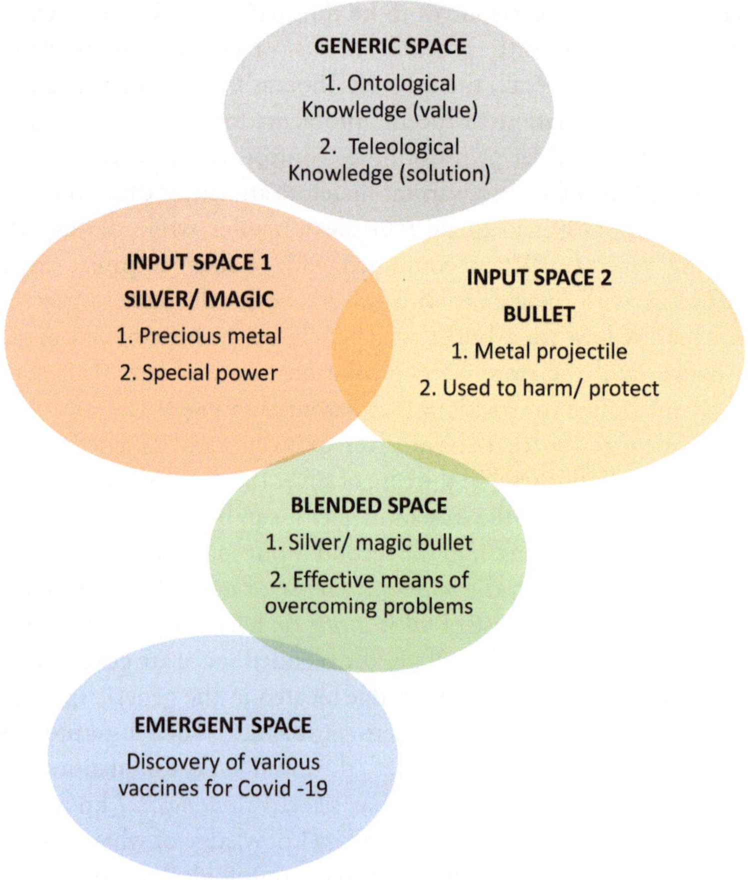

GENERIC SPACE
1. Ontological Knowledge (value)
2. Teleological Knowledge (solution)

INPUT SPACE 1
SILVER/ MAGIC
1. Precious metal
2. Special power

INPUT SPACE 2
BULLET
1. Metal projectile
2. Used to harm/ protect

BLENDED SPACE
1. Silver/ magic bullet
2. Effective means of overcoming problems

EMERGENT SPACE
Discovery of various vaccines for Covid -19

Fig. 9.1 'Silver/magic bullet' as a conceptual blend

In the 1930s a theory of communication known as 'Magic Bullet Theory' developed alongside 'Hypodermic Needle Theory' as two equally vivid metaphors to describe the effect of media communication on the public mind. It was argued that the media could project, or 'fire', a message or 'bullet', directly into the audience's mind and therefore was a 'magic bullet'. It was strongly influenced by behaviourism as it attributed an entirely passive role to the audience. The most well-known evidence in support of Magic Bullet Theory was an incident in 1938 when a radio broadcast of HG Wells's *War of the Worlds* in the style of a newscast led to widespread panic in the US as people genuinely believed it to be a true account of an alien invasion: these people had allowed the elephant of intuition to take over from the rider. The naming of the theory as 'Magic Bullet Theory' indicates the ongoing appeal of pre-modern notions of 'magic', as well as the attraction of metaphor in the naming of abstract ideas.

Thomas argues that during the sixteenth and seventeenth centuries English people, inspired by their Protestant theology, developed a self-confidence in their ability to overcome the hindrances they faced and removed the need for magic. So magic was a stop-gap solution that, for a period of time, co-existed with the rise of science. In examining the rhetorical power of appeals to magic, we should consider first whether the context activates a child or an adult frame and then the perspective which the 'magic' frame assumes: is it that of the magician, or of the supplicant? And what is the intention and role of the magician: is it the malign, exploitative magic of the quack doctor, the innocent magic of the wise healer, or the entertaining magic of the illusionist? 'Bullet' activates an adult frame of weapons, but when a speaker wants to present a policy as fantastical and beyond what is feasible, 'magic' may trigger a childish frame. This is all the more so with the phrase '*magic wand*': when asked about the shortage of personal protection equipment, Mr. Hancock told the Commons Health Committee.

I would love to be able to *wave a magic wand* and have PPE[9] fall from the sky in large quantities and be able to answer your question about when shortages will be resolved. But given that we have a global situation in which there is less PPE in the world than the world needs, obviously it's going to be a huge pressure point.[10]

Here Hancock implies that it is unrealistically childish to expect sufficient amounts of PPE. When Keir Starmer asked Boris Johnson what he would do to support firms faced with the financial impact of the pandemic Johnson replied:

We cannot, I'm afraid, simply with *a magic wand* ensure that every single job that was being done before the crisis is retained after the crisis.[11]

The reply was widely quoted in the press and on LBC radio a caller introduced as 'Mike from Harwich' used the same metaphor to criticise Keir Starmer for even asking Boris Johnson this question:

> He doesn't have the benefit of hindsight or *a magic wand*, he is doing his best.

It seems the 'magic wand' phrase convinced the caller of the impossibility of the government doing more to assist, and the expression 'waving a magic wand' implies that it is unreasonable to expect a solution: whatever is having a magic wand waved at it is represented as beyond the realm of the feasible in an adult world. Although the perspective is that of the magician, it introduces a fantasy image schema of a child dressed up in a wizard's outfit, or a Harry Potter costume, casting a spell.

A similar emphasis on the deceptiveness of 'simple' solutions that occurs in the phrase 'no silver bullet' is found in 'no magic bullet': it rejects solutions on the grounds that they are *too* simple. The 'no magic bullet' trope is a way of deflecting blame from the topical subject as it argues that there is simply nothing that experts can currently offer that provides a 'quick fix', or deceptively easy solution. 'Magic bullet' occurs in 315 news reports in the year from 1st March 2020, 'not a magic bullet' occurs in 81 of these reports and 'no magic bullet' occurs in 51 of them. In these cases, 'magic bullet' contributes to a counter argument that rejects solutions on the grounds they are *too* simple. The speaker warns against masquerading solutions and 'no magic bullet' can be described as creating a 'deceptively simple solution' frame. The use of this warrant is a way for the speaker to establish ethical credibility by creating an impression that a political or organisational spokesperson is only concerned with genuine *adult*, solutions rather than childish ones. The World Health Organization declared that vaccines are *no magic bullet* for the coronavirus crisis[12] though the phrase had already become a general refrain:

> Professor Louise Kenny, the pro vice chancellor for the faculty of health and life sciences at the University of Liverpool, warned there was *no 'magic bullet'* test with a one hundred per cent success rate. 'We *haven't got a magic test* but what we do have is a very helpful public intervention here,' she said.[13]

We're guessing some time in June we may get the results," said Prof Horby. "If it is really clear that there are benefits, an answer will be available quicker." But he warned that in the case of Covid-19, there would be *no magic bullet*.[14]

Jerome Adams, whose post makes him the operational head … went on to tell the Meet the Press programme on NBC News that there was *no magic bullet* or *magic cure* for coronavirus.[15]

It is ironic that the expression 'no magic bullet' implies that in other cases there might be a 'magic bullet', so rather than rejecting magic as the basis for knowledge, experts argue that there is no easy remedy in this particular case. The same is the case with 'magic formula", a public health professor was quoted in *The Sunday Times*:

So is Covid-19 still the killer it used to be? Or are we fumbling our way towards a *magic formula* of precautions, treatments and future vaccines that will turn this coronavirus from existential threat into manageable nuisance?[16]

The Australian Prime Minister Scott Morrison warned that:

no country has found *the magic formula* to this yet but Australia is better placed than most and many because of the strong position we went to this end.

So 'magic' does not in itself imply that a solution is impossible, sometimes we can achieve an unintended outcome, as can occur in scientific experimentation, but it implies that it is dishonest to have expectations that are *too* great and the potential of magic to activate either realistic 'adult' or impossible 'childish' hopes, valid or invalid moral intuitions, depends on the context. Another expression that occurred mostly in the negative but within an adult frame was 'magic pill':

The bad news is that there is *no magic pill* or *miracle broth* that will '*boost*' our immunity against coronavirus overnight.[17]

We were constantly crying and knackered and you want to do something but you can't go and see him, you can't make it better, can't take it away or give him *a magic pill*. There's physically nothing you can do and you feel so out of control, it was awful.[18]

However, when seeking to inspire enthusiasm and child-like optimism Boris Johnson was quite happy to put on his wizard's hat in a quest to evoke the childhood schema for magic, as in this speech in Dudley after the first wave and just before the first Lockdown was about to end:

We need now to *distil* the very best of the *psychic energy* of the last few months. Let's take the *zap* and *élan* of the armed services who helped to *build* the Nightingales. Let's take the selflessness and the love of the health and the care workers and the charities, the public spirit and the good humour of the entire population and let's *brew* them together with the *superhuman* energy of Captain Tom *bounding* around his garden at the age of 100 and raising millions for charity let's take that combination, that *spirit bottle* it, *swig* it and I believe we will have found if not quite *a magic potion*, at least the right *formula* to *get us through* these *dark* times.[19]

Here mixed metaphors proliferate and the scenario of brewing is blended with the supernatural to suggest magical power that can harness the forces of nature. Johnson prides himself on his ability to appeal to the elephant of moral intuition. The first-person plural ('we', 'us'), suggests that there is no longer a divide between magician and supplicant: this is more like a séance: an action invoking an elderly symbol of wise leadership in the shape of Captain Tom, a 100-year-old war veteran who raised money for the NHS by walking up and down his garden with his walking frame. Figure 9.2 shows how magic related compounds ('magic pills', 'magic wands' etc.) can be analysed as conceptual blends:

In these conceptual blends we have 'magic' in input space 1 which activates a schema for the supernatural and the power to influence events, in input space 2 there is various apparatus associated with magic—'wands', 'potions' etc.—all of which are instruments that can be used to protect (the idea of harm is suppressed in these blends, though is potentially there). From the generic space there is the knowledge of means and

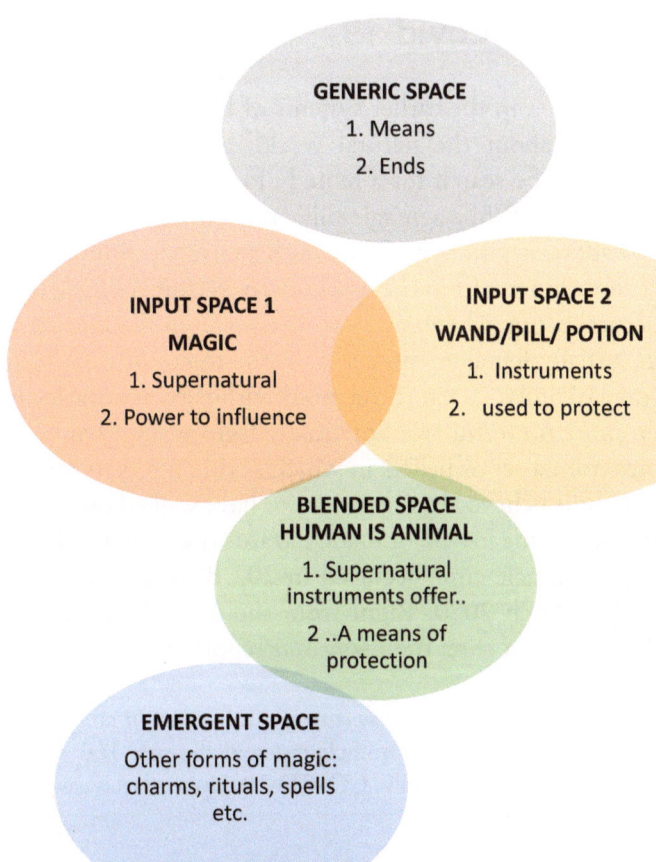

GENERIC SPACE
1. Means
2. Ends

INPUT SPACE 1
MAGIC
1. Supernatural
2. Power to influence

INPUT SPACE 2
WAND/PILL/ POTION
1. Instruments
2. used to protect

BLENDED SPACE
HUMAN IS ANIMAL
1. Supernatural instruments offer..
2 ..A means of protection

EMERGENT SPACE
Other forms of magic: charms, rituals, spells etc.

Fig. 9.2 'Magic' 'wand', 'pill', 'potion' etc. as a conceptual blend

ends, in political contexts this refers to the various range of alternative policy options for achieving political objectives. These drive the blend to arrive at the sense of a 'supernatural means of protection' in the blended space. In the emergent space are other means of performing magic such as chants, spells and rituals. Pragmatics determines whether these metaphor warrants are used negatively, or with a particular style such as irony, and therefore how they evaluate moral intuitions regarding Honesty and Dishonesty.

Miracle Cures for Covid-19

While magic originates in the earlier systems of belief deriving from traditional knowledge about the natural world, another metaphor that occurred to describe the search for a remedy for Covid-19 was the concept of a 'miracle cure'. While a 'magic pill' and 'a miracle cure' might be considered nowadays as synonyms, they do have rather different origins because 'miracle' originates from the power derived from a divine (usually male) supernatural being, whereas 'magic' derives from the knowledge of a wise person (usually female) who activates the forces of nature, rather than relying on a divinity. Given its religious authority, a 'miracle cure' is therefore even more powerful and potentially legitimising than a 'magic pill' as it comes from a set of beliefs in which divine intervention is possible, as when Jesus is believed by Christians to have walked on water, and to have transformed some loaves, or made Lazarus rise from his deathbed.

The expression 'miracle cure' occurred in 202 British press reports in the year from 1st March 2020. Right from the start of the crisis there were people looking for a cure; the *Daily Star* reported:

> Catholic shrine Lourdes closes '*miracle cure*' pools because of coronavirus; The site, which claims 69 verified miracle cures in the past 160 years, is taking no chances with the deadly COVID-19 virus that is sweeping the globe.[20]

The usual charlatans that any crisis invites were quick to be trying to exploit the situation:

> A British man has been charged with a federal crime after being accused of smuggling a phoney coronavirus cure into the US, prosecutors said.
>
> Frank Richard Ludlow of West Sussex was charged in Los Angeles federal court with introducing misbranded drugs into interstate commerce and could face up to three years in prison if convicted, according to the US attorney's office. Mr. Ludlow is in custody after being arrested on drug charges in the UK last week. Prosecutors alleged that Mr. Ludlow, who is not a doctor, had been selling a concoction called "Trinity Remedy", that he touted as a "*miracle cure*" for various ailments, to people in California and Utah via mail.[21]

A California doctor has been charged with fraud for allegedly selling "Covid-19 Treatment Packs" he claimed could be a *"miracle cure"* for people who contract the novel virus. ... When speaking to the undercover FBI agent, Dr Staley allegedly described the medication as a "miracle cure" that would cure "100 per cent" of the novel virus.[22]

In these examples 'miracle cure' appears in scare quotes suggesting that it is employed sarcastically by the journalist. Some of these 'snake oil salesmen' were motivated by greed while others by gratification of an inherent narcissism. A religious leader, Mark Grenon, wrote a letter to Donald Trump stating that chlorine dioxide—a powerful bleach—is "a wonderful detox that can kill 99% of the pathogens in the body" and "can rid the body of Covid-19".[23] Grenon was arrested along with his son in April 2020 and in the same month an American man died from self-medicating with chloroquine. Why should a religious leader be giving advice in areas where he has no professional expertise? One explanation is that some religious figures resented the legitimacy attributed to scientists during a pandemic because they view science itself as a challenge to their authority; they compete for the role of rider of the elephant! In an article for *The Guardian* Ed Pilkington used a number of metaphors (in italics), some his own and others in the reported speech of American scientists:

Three months into the pandemic, with the number of confirmed cases passing 1 million, the tension that *has been simmering* for months between Trump and the scientific world *is at boiling point.* His improvisation about injecting disinfectant *encapsulated* the sense of demoralization—of despair, almost—that many American scientists now feel about the *drift* from evidence-based leadership.

"They are doing everything they can to *undermine* science at a time when it is critically important, as are facts. We have come to an extreme level," said Gina McCarthy, who led the US Environmental Protection Agency (EPA) until Trump's accession in 2017. Science is *so assailed* at present that the situation raises a startling question: are we *losing the fight* for reason in the pandemic? McCarthy ... said she frets America may prove incapable of withstanding the anti-science *assault unleashed* by Trump."[24]

In the first sentence the metaphors derive conceptually from ANGER IS HOT FLUID IN A CONTAINER to describe the emotional intensity of the debate between American scientists and Trump; in the second paragraph they are from the semantic field of war and conflict to bring a sense of urgency to the struggle between two ideologies: 'Science' and 'Christian Evangelism'. Pilkington then summarises the argument, for which he has demonstrated support among scientists, that Trump is ideologically opposed to science:

> In Trump Republicans have found a leader who regards his own innate abilities to *divine the truth* as superior to evidence-based science. In one of the most telling moments of his daily White House coronavirus briefings, Trump was asked what metrics he would use to decide when Americans could *emerge* from lockdown.
>
> He raised his right hand, placed his index finger against his temple, and said: "The metrics right here. That's my metrics."
>
> That faith in his own instincts over and above fact has been a characteristic for years. Trump is famous for believing that exercise is misguided, because *people are born with a finite amount of energy in them, like batteries*. ... Trump was slow to *mobilise* the federal government because he failed to *heed* scientific warnings; instead he chose to *follow* his "hunch" that a "*miracle*" would happen and the virus would disappear.[25]

'Divine the truth' introduces a schema for magical insight as in 'water divination' and Trump's faith in his own moral intuition rather than empiricism is expressed by the gestural metaphor of pointing to his head (often a gesture to indicate craziness). The prioritisation of individual insight over shared group understanding is a characteristic of the narcissistic personality: one for whom the rider of reason is rarely in control. Here metaphor is employed by the journalist to determine his selection of quotations from scientists, from Donald Trump and also to summarise his own criticism of the ideology he attributes to Trump. His evaluation of Trump is based on the moral frame of Honesty and Dishonesty: he states that Trump's views are not based on science and implies that they are fundamentally Dishonest.

The extensive use of metaphor in argument is shared by other journalists keen to undermine the appeal of 'miracle cures' and undermine the legitimacy of their ideological opponents in a 'no holds barred' rhetoric that emphasises the fundamental Dishonesty and false thinking about the Covid-19 pandemic. In a powerful, emotional article that seeks to explain the basis of conspiracy theories Noah Berlatsky states:

> *Quack* cures are lies—and lies are *the fuel that powers* the right in the United States. … *Selling snake oil* and *selling bigotry* are not that different. They both rely on a contempt for one's audience and a contempt for the truth. *Peddling* hatred requires a *near-constant stream* of untruths and conspiracy theories, big and small: black people aren't intelligent; Jews are plotting to undermine the white race; trans women lurk in bathrooms to assault cis women. To get people to buy prejudice and *quack* cures alike, you have to *pry your marks away* from the *solid land* of fact and set them loose on a *sea of bilge* and nonsense.
>
> Fascists and *snake oil salesman* are not just *peddling* lies, though. They're *peddling secret knowledge*, and *entry into a club*, or *an inner circle*. The appeal of the *supplement* you can purchase exclusively is much the same as the appeal of the conspiracy theory that lets you know that George Soros, or Barack Obama, or the Jews, or the Chinese, are the true *enemy*. To believe in hydroxychloroquine or white supremacy is to believe that *you are among the elect*. The appeal of believing a lie is that you end up certain of a truth that belongs to a *besieged* epistemological minority.[26]

In the first paragraph there is a blending of selling snake oil and selling bigotry, this is then developed with a frame of unreliable knowledge as water ('stream', 'bilge') and reliable knowledge as 'land'. In the next paragraph metaphors are based on spatial deixis in which there is a 'container', where those who are close to the speaker, and to purported truth, form an 'inner circle'. Here the perspective of the metaphors shifts from that of the author, who views purveyors of miracle cures as snake oil salesmen, to that of the represented agent, Trump—the perpetrator of Dishonesty. The war frame appears in 'enemy' and 'besieged' to reinforce a 'them' versus 'us' construal. It is through his metaphors that the writer, Noah Berlatsky, shows emotional commitment to the moral intuitions of his position: he rejects 'miracle cures' as undermining morality by contributing to Harm and Cheating, but, above all because they are Dishonest, as implied by 'snake oil salesman'. There is also the moral intuition of

Disgust in the image of 'a sea of bilge': rhetorically, his arguments are intensified and empowered by using metaphors to appeal to a range of moral intuitions.

I decided to get an idea of the diversity and frequency of 'miracle cure' stories in the British press by examining the number of stories that used the phrase 'miracle cure' when referring to a particular *type* of miracle cure (e.g. 'chloroquine') over a one year period from 1st March 2020; the results are summarised in Table 9.1:

Of course, 'miracle cures' were part of a wider discourse of misinformation that included diverse conspiracy theories ranging from the claim that Bill Gates was hatching a scheme to inject microchips to track and control people, or that it was a cover for a takeover by artificial intelligence, and that 5G technology was causing the spread of coronavirus. These stories often profiled the role of celebrities in spreading the conspiracy theory via their own social media channels. Some research shows that conspiracy theories can be related to the dangers of vaccines, from common feelings of powerlessness, disillusionment and mistrust in authorities; it also showed that "participants who had been exposed to material supporting anti-vaccine conspiracy theories showed less intention to vaccinate than those in the anti-conspiracy condition or controls".[27] There were conspiracy theories more specifically related to divisions within US politics, for example that it was a plot by the 'deep state' supported by the Democratic Party to establish a new world order and, in foreign policy, or that SARS-CoV-2 had leaked from a secret bioweapons facility in Wuhan or originated from humans consuming bats in Wuhan. Metaphor was employed by journalists who, by appealing to the moral intuition of Honesty and Dishonesty, exposed and condemned such misinformation and its perpetrators.

The 'Race' for a Vaccine

The only 'magic' that science could offer for Covid-19 was a vaccine against the disease and this was commonly thought of in terms of a competitive race, first between scientists and Covid-19, then as a race between different laboratories to develop a vaccine, and then, once a vaccine had been developed, as a race between different countries to obtain the

Table 9.1 Types of 'miracle cure' reported in the British Press (2020–2021)

Type of 'miracle cure' or 'magic'	Example	No, of reports
Drinking alcohol	Why alcohol is a blow to your immune system and YOU should avoid drinking it if getting the Covid-19 vaccine	167
Chloroquine or hydorxychloroquine	During his daily coronavirus press briefings, the president has repeatedly plugged the use of hydroxychloroquine as a miracle cure for the deadly virus.	146
Use of salt or saline	Incorrect claims widely shared include that Covid-19 could be alleviated by gargling salt water Saline rinse and mouthwash can help prevent infection	112
5G	WhatsApp tries to slow the spread of viral messages, such as the theory that coronavirus is linked to 5G.	53
Saying a prayer	Consumers were instructed to add 18 ounces of water, say a prayer, drink half of the solution, take a probiotic along with bee pollen, and then ingest the remainder of the solution, said prosecutors.	49
Eating garlic	However, there is "no evidence from the current outbreak that eating garlic has protected people from the new coronavirus", says the WHO.	33
Taking cocaine	Starting off the back of promising developments, cocaine became a "miracle cure" that could treat anything from toothache to depression.	29
Drinking urine	Unlike many other past remedies that have died out, urine drinking is still practiced by far-out "alternative medicine" practitioners.	13
Drinking mineral solution	The substance, chlorine dioxide, is a powerful bleach used in textile manufacturing. The Grenons market it as "miracle mineral solution" or MMS which they say when drunk as a dilution can cure almost all illnesses including Covid, cancer, HIV/aids as well as the condition autism.	11

vaccine, and finally as a race to inoculate the population against the disease. So there were several types of race: a bioscientific race between scientists and Covid-19, an economic race between different research laboratories, Astra Zeneca, Pfizer etc., each of which was seeking to develop an effective vaccine and a political race between different nations as they sought to obtain and distribute the vaccine. This was because once a vaccine had been discovered there was a race between the spread of the disease amongst those who were not immune and the implementation of an effective vaccine programme that could reach these people. There were, then, a series of interlinking and partially simultaneous races all of which profiled the importance of time because without the implementation of a vaccine programme in record-breaking time, national health systems were reaching a situation beyond their control. For this reason, a Competitive Race frame was frequently used to articulate the moral frame of Care and Harm: without a vaccine all would be lost. Table 9.2 illustrates a range of words and phrases from the semantic field of competitive race that occurred frequently in the media and in the language of politicians:

The competitive Race frame had been well established and has an ideological motivation because it originated in the tendency of global capitalism to represent politics as a 'race' of nations seeking to outperform their 'competitors'. These derived from neo-Darwinist outlooks that view human progress as some sort of struggle for survival in which those nations that have greater access to vaccines are much better 'equipped' for survival. The neo-liberal concept of the 'global race' originated in the earlier political concept of nations being involved in an 'arms race' and later a more positive prosody for 'race' began to emerge in the metaphor of the 'space race'—whose original reference was to the competition to put a man on the moon. The 'global race' metaphor dominated in the period of globalization during the 1990's by both New Labour and then was picked up on my David Cameron and more recently in Boris Johnson's notion of 'global Britain'. However, unlike purely economic interpretations of the Competitive Race frame, there was a greater Darwinian emphasis in this frame in relation to the development of a vaccine for Covid-19 since it seemed a real possibility that there could be a 'zombie apocalypse' if a vaccine was not developed and might result in the collapse of health systems worldwide. This was a race that you

Table 9.2 Competitive Race metaphors and the vaccine in the British Press (2020–2021)

Pace	Limited supply of the two approved COVID-19 vaccines has hampered the *pace* of vaccinations—and that was before extreme winter weather delayed the delivery of about 6 million doses this past week. (*The Independent*, 21 February 2021)	3416
Accelerate	To hit this ambitious target it will have to *accelerate* its vaccine programme at breakneck speed to hit an average 2million per week, including this week … The MHRA, is also to increase staffing in a bid to *accelerate* the mass vaccination programme (*MailOnline*, 7 January 2021)	2068
Catch up	The progress of the Novavax vaccine represents another success for the UK's Vaccines Task Force, which has left the EU scrambling to *catch up*. A sluggish regulatory process in Brussels has meant only the Pfizer vaccine has so far been approved for use in the EU. (*MailOnline*, 29 January 2021)	1273
Fast track	Britain 'will be first' to get doses of Oxford University's Covid-19 vaccine if it works, Number 10 confirmed today amid claims Donald Trump is aiming to *fast-track* the experimental vaccine into use before the US election this autumn. (*MailOnline*, 24 August 2020)	684
Sluggish	Brussels has been under growing pressure from member states over its *sluggish* vaccine programme, which has seen inoculations fall far behind the UK (*MailOnline*, 29 January 2021)	449
Track record	Have hope—the UK has a *track record* of successful vaccine campaigns (*The Guardian*, 30 November 2020)	364
Sprint	'Substantial ramp-up in second *sprint* for vaccines, says NHS boss. (*telegraph.co.uk*, 15 February 2021)	357
Race against time	AS THE COUNTRY and the world awaits a coronavirus vaccine, *a race against time* to conduct human trials has emerged due to the decline of Covid-19 infections in the UK. (*Express Online*, 31 May 2020) This is a *race against time* to vaccinate the vulnerable (*The Times*, 5 January 2021)	289
Overtake	We may have gained a head start in rolling out vaccines, but other countries are starting to *overtake* us.	202
High speed	The paper suggested that even a *high-speed* vaccine *rollout* reaching 3.2million doses per week—2.5 m were administered last week—may only lead to two thirds of the country developing immunity by the middle of summer. (*MailOnline*, 22 February 2021)	163

(continued)

Table 9.2 (continued)

Lag behind/ laggard	Timeline of virus vaccine deals reveals EU's *lag behind*. (*The Independent* 7 February 2021) The government had rejected accusations of being a *vaccine laggard*, saying high levels of resistance to the jabs in France required a cautious approach. (*MailOnline*, 17 January 2021)	183
Relay race	'The bad news is that fighting covid has been from the beginning a *relay race*: everybody has to do their piece for everybody else to do their piece, and *the baton has been dropped by the runner … handling it in the final leg.*' (Peter Pitts, former FDA official). (*MailOnline*, 31 December 2020)	85
Tortoise	Even the *tortoise*—like European Medicines Agency has now decided the Oxford/AstraZeneca vaccine is suitable for use on all age groups. *telegraph.co.uk* (3 February 2021)	50

could not afford to opt out of, and although it reinforced the conceptual metaphor NATION STATES ARE COMPETITORS it also had the potential to encourage the notion that humanity is in a race against other potential and related sources of destruction such as the climate crisis. To the extent that the Competitive Race frame motivated governments and scientists to develop a vaccine, health systems to distribute this vaccine, and people to come forward to be inoculated it was a valid frame for politicians and opinion formers alike. In the same way that 'war' metaphors could stimulate action, so the Competitive Race frame heightened a psychological climate of emergency.

Metaphoric Thought in Pro- and Anti-Vaccine Discourse

As we saw in the first section of this chapter, one of the 'silver' or 'magic' 'bullets' was the development of a vaccine for Covid-19; there were 522 news reports in the year from 1st March 2020 that included both 'silver bullet' and 'vaccine' or 'magic bullet' and 'vaccine' (we will recall that there were over 1000 reports with one or other of these expressions—so there were other types of 'silver/ magic' 'bullet). Right from the start there were warnings against over-optimism about vaccines:

In any case, vaccines might not be the *magic bullet* we think.

However, scientists tell us that the coronavirus is here to stay and we may face new strains of it, so a vaccine is no *silver bullet*.

But the idea of a vaccine—the *silver bullet* quintessential—has come to bear an almost unreasonable allure.

Even when research had produced a range of vaccines by early 2021 the same metaphors still expressed a degree of caution:

But SAGE experts warned in a later briefing today that, although the vaccine results are promising, they are not a *silver bullet*.

There 'might never be a *silver bullet* treatment' for the coronavirus pandemic, the World Health Organisation WHO has warned.

He (Lord Sumption) added: "It will not be a *magic bullet*.

Can you hear it? Is that the beautiful sound of a *silver bullet* whistling our way? Though the prime minister does not "want to get people's hopes up" he suggests it is "possible that we will make significant progress on the vaccine this year".

It is not surprising that 'bullet' metaphors were widely used to report on vaccine development because the vaccine had long been construed as a 'weapon'. There were 6262 reports in which 'weapon' occurred within 5 words of vaccine as in the following:

He (Matt Hancock) said: "This is positive news and, if approved by the medicines regulator, the Novavax vaccine will be a significant boost to our vaccination programme and another *weapon* in our *arsenal* to beat this awful virus."[28]

...senior German MEP who called for the EU to "show our *weapons*" in a vaccine trade *war*.[29]

Evidence suggests the Oxford University vaccine—the main *weapon* in Britain's *arsenal* to *combat* the virus—does not stop people falling ill with the South African variant.[30]

Even among those opposed to the war frame for Covid they rarely cited 'weapon' as an example, perhaps because the notion of weapon implies the ability to destroy a virus that was indisputably harmful to mankind, therefore, to reject the 'weapon' metaphor would be indirectly encouraging the virus to spread by removing its major threat. Unlike some other 'weapons' there was little risk of 'collateral damage'. This is an illustration of how the priming of a semantic field by metaphors like 'silver bullet' can pave the way for later conceptualisations of the vaccine as a 'weapon', as in the following:

> NHS Test and Trace is a crucial *weapon* against this virus, but it is not a *silver bullet*.[31]

> While the vaccine developments are extremely encouraging, medical interventions alone are unlikely to provide a *silver bullet* in the near-term. Science is one of our most potent *weapons* in this fight.[32]

Politicians were keen to harness the persuasive power of metaphor to the goals of encouraging the take-up of the vaccine. As *The Times* reported Boris Johnson as saying:

> We have talked for a long time, or I have, about *the distant bugle of the scientific cavalry coming over the brow of the hill*. And tonight that *toot of the bugle is louder*. But it is still some way off.[33]

> Mass testing and the vaccine are *vital arrows in our epidemiological quiver*.[34]

> I remain buoyantly optimistic about the prospects of this country next year. I just don't want to let people run away with the idea that this development is today is necessarily *a home run, a slam dunk, a shot to the back of the net*, yet.[35]

Here three completely different frames are activated for an identical purpose of encouraging optimism about the vaccine; the first is a rather ethno-centric frame from a 1960s western of last minute rescue by the intervention of the cavalry; in the second it is still a bows and arrows one, but not the arrows of native American Indians but an archery lawn in Surrey, and in the third he curiously draws on metaphors from American sports before introducing a British one, probably seeking to ally himself with the new American President, Joe Biden.

The Deputy Chief Medical Officer, Jonathan Van-Tam also developed a reputation for framing the vaccine with colourful metaphors again from completely different frames; in the extended metaphors below, the first is from a football penalty shoot-out frame, the second from the journey frame:

> This is like … getting to the end of the play-off final, it's gone to penalties, the first player goes up and scores goal. You haven't won the cup yet, but what it does is it tells you that the goalkeeper can be beaten.[36]

It is unquestionable that anyone should not want their team to win a final in a penalty shoot-out and it puts the pro-vaccine lobby as on the side that is taking the penalty—the reader-hearer perspective and the role of the virus in that of the opposing team that had previously been viewed as insuperable but had now been shown not to be invincible. A similar argument is implied by activating the journey frame:

> This, to me, is like a train journey where you're standing on the station— it's wet, windy, it's horrible—and two miles down the tracks, two lights appear and it's the train. And it's a long way off. We're at that point at the moment. That's the efficacy result. Then we hope the train slows down safely to get into the station. That the safety data. And then the train stops. And at that point the doors don't open. The guard has to make sure it's safe to open the doors. That's the MHRA [Medicines and Healthcare products Regulatory Agency], that's the regulator. And, when the doors open, I hope there's not an unholy scramble for the seats. The JCVI [joint committee on vaccination and immunisation] has very clearly said which people are going to need the seats most and they are the ones who should get on the train first.[37]

In this metaphor, it has become an allegory for correct behaviour, which takes for granted the idea that everyone will want to get onto the train, so taking a vaccine is as purposeful as taking a rail journey, something almost routine and certainly not where risk-calculations are usually made. The idea of there being not enough seats on the train for everyone to get one draws on the familiar experience of train travel and argues that the vaccine is in short supply, as train seats are, so there is the implication that if you are offered a vaccine don't miss your chance as another way may not come along soon. Framing by metaphor is something characteristic of the communication style of both speakers and they clearly contain implied arguments and evaluations concerning the efficacy, and safety of the vaccine.

This is not the only 'journey' metaphor that he uses, as when discussing the strong possibility of a vaccine being discovered in the near future he employed a 'flight' metaphor:

> Turning to a flight metaphor, Prof Van Tam added: "Do I believe we're now on the glide path to landing this plane Yes, I think I do. "Do I accept that sometimes when you're on the glide path you can have a side wind and the landing is not totally straightforward—of course. "And this is the real science world we live in. But yes, I think we're on the glide path. "Over."[38]

To some extent Van-Tam was concerned simply to reinforce the 'journey' frame because, as we saw earlier, the government's policy for ending the Lockdown was framed as 'the roadmap'; this term was used in 1376 different news stories in the UK press in the year from 1st March 2020, whereas it was only used in 91 reports in the preceding year. So when Van-Tam employed the journey frame he was reinforcing the preferred frame of government communication.

By contrast, those who were opposed to the vaccine were also quick to employ metaphors they thought would enforce their arguments. On twitter they frequently posted the sheep icon to argue that uncritical acceptance of the vaccine was simply following others. Anti-vaxxer frames sort to address the beliefs and concerns of minority audiences who might be especially amenable to such narratives; these included conspiracy theorists concerned about the global power of 'Big Pharma' who might be aiming to control population. There were various multi-ethnic communities who were anxious about vaccines: a study from the Royal Society for Public Health found 57% of BAME people said they would take the vaccine compared with

79% of white people. Some Muslim religious groups were concerned about the purity of the vaccine. Another group who had cause for concern were younger women who were anxious about the effects on their fertility or on an unborn child. These doubts probably increased after they were identified as being at risk of blood clots from the Astra Zeneca vaccine. Other groups who were 'hesitant' about vaccine were some workers who were first in line to receive the vaccination; these included care-home workers and NHS staff some of whom believed that they were being treated as guinea-pigs: there was no shortage of the elephant of intuition anywhere.

In the United States, Dr. Anthony Fauci was accused by conspiracists of exaggerating deaths or being a beneficiary of pharmaceutical efforts to find treatments and a vaccine. Social media shares of these reports were often combined with popular hashtags such as #FireFauci and #FauciFraud. Some national leaders were opposed to the vaccine from the start. In Tanzania, President Magufuli who had become president in 2015, was nicknamed "The Bulldozer" because of his reputation for getting things done. In January 2021 he said:

> The Ministry of Health should be careful, they should not hurry to try these vaccines without doing research, not every vaccine is important to us, we should be careful. We should not be used as *'guinea pigs'*.

He warned that:

> Vaccinations are dangerous. If the white man was able to come up with vaccinations, he should have found a vaccination for Aids, cancer and TB by now. In place of searching for a vaccine people should concentrate on saying prayers and using traditional medicine such as steam inhalation,[39]

Sadly, John Magufuli died on 17 March 2021 at the age of 61. It is supposed that the cause of his death was Covid-19, but as his government no longer kept records, this cannot be confirmed.

There was nothing new about many of the fears of those who were opposed to vaccinations; ever since Edward Jenner experimented by injecting a boy with lymph from the blister of a milkmaid infected with cowpox to find a vaccine for smallpox, there had been concern that this was not a Christian practice because it disrupted the natural order by putting animal matter into the human body. The mandatory vaccination of infants up to 3 months old in 1853 led parents to fear they had lost control over their children's bodies and this led to the formation of the Anti-Vaccination League and the Anti-Compulsory Vaccination League and a range of anti-vaccination journals. The fact that there were *two* leagues is significant because the original opponents were opposed to the principle of vaccination itself, whereas it subsequently became the idea of *compulsory* vaccination as an infringement of human liberty that took over. In 1885 between 80 and 100,000 people attended an anti-vaccine march in Leicester which became the focal point of the movement.

I would like to suggest that metaphoric thinking underlay many of the moral intuitions of the original nineteenth century opposition to vaccination: while both humans and animals had bodies, humans were in control of their bodies whereas animals were subject to the control of humans, to reverse this would be to disrupt the natural order. Human bodies were naturally, intuitively, clean and therefore healthy, whereas animal bodies were typically dirty and diseased, so the intuition arose that inserting something from a diseased animal body into a human would be likely to cause infection rather than to terminate it. The human body was sacrosanct and should not be violated by incisions, whereas the animal body was base, to treat a human body like an animal body by injecting puss would therefore violate its sanctity. This apparently literal blending of the human and the animal occurs in a cartoon of 1802 by James Gillray, with the ironic caption 'Wonderful Effects of Inoculation'. It can be viewed at: https://en.wikipedia.org/wiki/File:The_cow_pock.jpg and it depicts people with udders, horns etc. projecting from various parts of their body and is a highly satirical comment on the absurdity of the views on those opposed to vaccination; it is to be noted that the picture on the wall depicts the golden calf; it is analysed as a metaphor blend in Fig. 9.3.

From the anti-vaccine movement of the nineteenth century there was moral intuition that injection with decaying and diseased matter extracted from animals could have contaminating and degrading effects on humans and in 1920 Chas M. Higgins published a short book the 'Horrors of Vaccination Exposed and Illustrated'.[40] The case against vaccination is argued with conviction drawing on ethical and logical appeals and

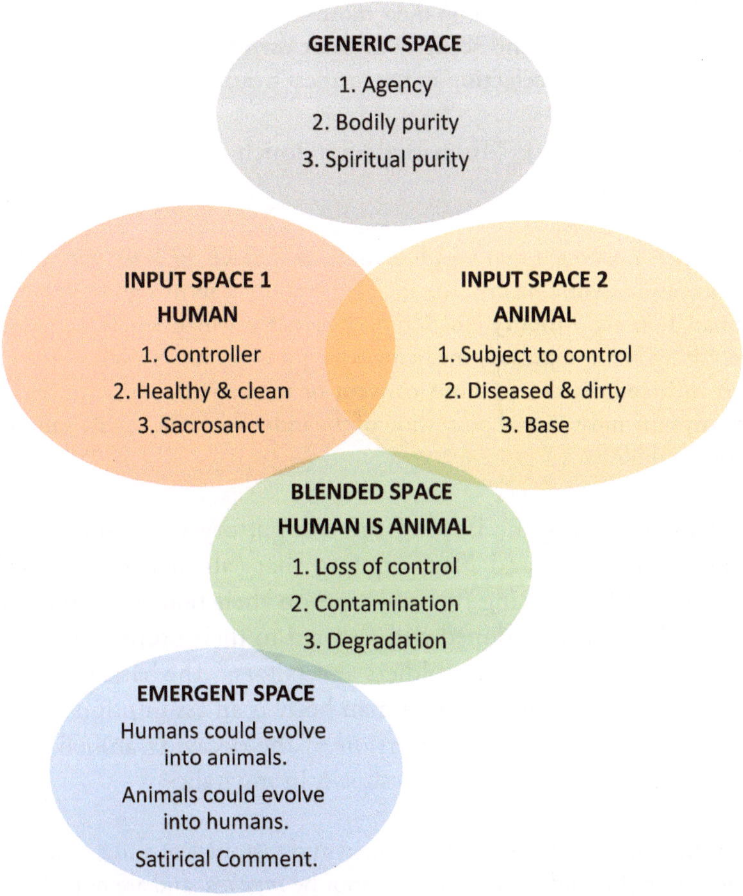

Fig. 9.3 Blending of human and animal in anti-vaccination metaphors

discusses the compulsory vaccination of those serving in the American armed forces. It is broad ranging in its moral arguments with appeals to a wide range of moral intuitions especially Liberty; he argues that it is an inalienable right to control what enters your body. He appeals to Care & Harm and the argument is supported by statistics showing that the risks of dying from vaccination exceed those of dying from smallpox. It makes particular appeals to the sanctity of the human body based on the moral intuition of Sanctity and Degradation:

Have the people ever given up their most sacred essential and unalienable right to **the sanctity and security of their own bodies** and to their **free choice and right of selection** in the medical treatment of their bodies?

Later he cites Plato: "Thou shalt not touch that which is mine" to develop an argument:

Thou shalt not touch that which is mine or remove the least thing which belongs to me without my consent," is certainly a most righteous rule of human honesty, **sanctity, justice** and **security** which surely condemns everything like compulsory medicine which touches and **violates** the body with **inflicted** disease, **without consent** of the patient, and removes and **destroys** the most **sacred** possession of the individual, viz. bodily **sanctity**, health and life.

He was addressing the issue of the compulsory vaccination of those serving in the Army and Navy arguing that "all men condemned by Court Martial for refusing the infliction on their bodies of compulsory disease shall be fully pardoned and restored to their proper and honourable status as loyal American soldiers and sailors." The basis for his arguments about the sanctity of the human body is an assumption of human purity and the intuition that insertion of the decaying animal into the healthy human is a degradation as shown in my italics:

Now, the true American ... are free men and members of a free state, with American rights and dignities that cannot be *invaded*, and are not "slaves," "chattels," or "subjects" to any one, and, therefore, are not to be treated by any form of military despotism or arbitrary medical dictation, *as slaves, hogs, or cattle* might be so treated.

Here he accuses despots as treating humans as if they were animals i.e. that they are making a category error of the same type as occurs in metaphor. He develops the metaphor with the equivalence of animal and human doctors:

And *as the hog or cattle* doctor might properly force any medicine down the throat of the helpless *beast* without being required to say "by your leave" to his humble *patient*, or might perform on the body of the helpless *animal* any operation that he or the owner might decide upon, yet I think that neither of us would admit that any *man* calling himself a *human* doctor could, with any decency, propriety, or legality, follow this crude but necessary code of ethics of the *animal doctor* on the *human* subject by attempting to perform any medical service on the *human* body by any intimidation or force or without **full approval and consent** of the patient.

It seems, above all, the intermingling of the human body with the animal body that invites the emotion of disgust and appeals to the moral intuition of Sanctity and Degradation:

it is obvious that the man is no longer a *sovereign* or the *owner* of his own body, but is a mere "*slave*" or *domestic animal* and that the doctor really *owns* his body and is his "*master*" as much as if he were a *pig* or *dog*; so that, therefore, all "equality" and "*sovereignty*" of the individual is destroyed by this medical "*hoggery*" and we have not a "government of the people, by the people, for the people," but a government of the doctors, by the doctors, for the doctors, which in fact we now have to a very dangerous extent.

Here he blends the ideas of human and animal knowledge with the neologism 'hoggery' as if medical experts are themselves behaving like animals in advocating something that not only denies individual liberties but does so in a way that is both dangerous and disgusting! Ultimately, it is the practice itself that revolts him as going intuitively against nature:

We must never forget that vaccination is an evil. Vaccinia is just as much a disease as smallpox, though a less serious one, and all diseases must be regarded as evil and to be avoided, if possible. There is not the slightest evidence that vaccination, apart from its effect in preventing smallpox, is of the least value or anything but detrimental to the human race.

He does not rely greatly on metaphor, and, when he does, it is to a biblical metaphor for cause and effect within an ethical context:

Is it physically or medically possible to go on *sowing* and *spreading* some known and unknown septic diseases at whole sale within human bodies, without *reaping* some big *harvest* of deadly septic diseases as a necessary consequence? In the words of Scripture, can we keep on *"sowing" the "winds"* of infection without ultimately "reaping" the "whirlwind" of epidemics?

The sanctity of the human body, moral intuitions about injecting septic matter into a healthy person, and the dangers of it going wrong are all basic concerns that can be found today among anti-vaxxers and sometimes the vaccine-hesitant. These are not irrational beliefs, but they are ones that are based on moral intuitions alone; however, those who choose to get vaccinated, even when themselves not in a risk group, are also displaying a strong and valid ethical position based on the moral intuitions of Care for themselves and Fairness towards others and also on the rider of reason. A very powerful explanatory metaphor for the principle underlying vaccination is offered by Biss:if we imagine the action of a vaccine not just in terms of how it affects a single body, but also in terms of how it affects the collective body of a community, it is fair to think of vaccination as *a kind of banking of immunity. Contributions to this bank are donations* to those who cannot or will not be protected by their own immunity.[41]

In this argument it is more altruistic to get vaccinated since those who remain unvaccinated, while guarding the sanctity of their own bodies and avoiding the risk of side-effects, are also piggy-backing on the immunity of others who have chosen to get vaccinated. It is rather like an insurance system: insurance can *only* exist if a certain amount of people agree to pay into a central fund, even though they may not be the ones most likely to take withdrawals from this fund. The pooling of risk is a characteristic of an ethical society that has principles that reject the idea of each man for himself and let the devil take the hindmost. It is a moral intuition that seeks to put the rider of reason back in control of the elephant of intuition.

For both the opponents and supporters of vaccination, metaphor offers the potential for explanation by analogy (using prior knowledge) and increased emotional investment by arousing disgust or enthusiasm. There were opponents, who were following a historical pre-scientific tradition in their rejection of vaccines: we saw how Chas Higgins framed humans as in danger of losing their sanctity if injected with decaying animal matter. However, supporters of the vaccine expressed their enthusiasm for it in different ways: Gillray satirized vaccine opposition and vaccines were also framed in terms of other social arrangements such as banking and insurance that appeal to the moral intuition of Fairness and Honesty. In the current pandemic the Competitive Race frame is used to articulate the urgent need to develop a vaccine, obtain it and then distribute it among their populations to give them a better chance of survival based on moral intuitions concerning Care and Harm. Both pro- and anti-vaccine advocates therefore employ metaphor to establish and reinforce the moral intuitions of their respective arguments, but one seeks to restore the rider of reason while the other allows the elephant of intuition to rampage.

Notes

1. https://www.acampbell.org.uk/bookreviews/r/thomas-k.html. Accessed 26 June 2021.
2. *The Guardian*, 13 August 2020.
3. *The Guardian*, 26 January 2021.
4. *mirror.co.uk*, 3 August 2020.
5. *telegraph.co.uk*, 26 September 2020.
6. *mirror.co.uk*, 13 October 2020.
7. *MailOnline*, 6 September 2020.
8. *Express Online*, 20 December 2020.
9. 'PPE' refers to Personal Protective Equipment.
10. *mirror.co.uk*, 17 April 2020.
11. *MailOnline*, 15 July 2020.
12. *The Guardian,* 4 December 2020.
13. *MailOnline*, 23 December 2020.
14. *The Guardian*, 17 April 2020.
15. *The Guardian*, 5 April 2020.
16. *The Sunday Times*, 6 September 2020.
17. *MailOnline*, 14 March 2020.
18. *mirror.co.uk*, 9 May 2020.
19. https://www.gov.uk/government/speeches/pm-economy-speech-30-june-2020. Accessed 26 June 2021.
20. *Daily Star Online*, 4 March 2020.
21. *The Independent*, 2 April 2020.

22. *The Independent,* 19 April 2020.
23. *The Guardian,* 24 April 2020.
24. *The Guardian,* 3 May 2020.
25. *The Guardian,* 3 May 2020.
26. *The Independent (United Kingdom),* 19 May 2020.
27. https://doi.org/10.1371/journal.pone.0089177. Accessed 26 June 2021.
28. *Express Online,* 29 January 2021.
29. *The Times (London),* 30 January 2021.
30. *MailOnline,* 9 February 2021.
31. *MailOnline,* 9 November 2020.
32. *telegraph.co.uk,* 18 November 2020.
33. *The Times,* 10 November 2020.
34. *The Guardian,* 9 November 2020.
35. *The Guardian,* 9 November 2020.
36. *The Guardian,* 9 November 2020.
37. *The Guardian,* 9 November 2020.
38. *mirror.co.uk,* 20 November 2020.
39. BBC 27 January 2021
40. https://ia800704.us.archive.org/28/items/39002086340891.med.yale.edu/39002086340891.med.yale.edu.pdf. Accessed 26 June 2021.
41. Biss, E. (2014). *On Immunity: An Inoculation.*

10

Honesty and Dishonesty in Pandemic Language

One of the difficulties with advocating honesty as a moral intuition is that it sets rather a high standard on the advocate, and, to avoid hypocrisy, I should declare that I have not always been entirely candid in my own affairs hence the need at this finishing point for a confession. I recall a time when working in Morocco for a British company that I received my salary *twice* due to an accounting error: yes, not one but two salaries for the month: a banking error, for once, in my favour! This was just before a major football tournament, and I have to confess that I interpreted the banking error as a blessing as I needed to buy a colour television so as to watch this tournament. I had recently moved to Rabat, the capital city, and was particularly keen to watch the event. It was worth the purchase: Morocco beat Portugal 3–0 and the party went on all night. When queried about the double payment I denied having received the first payment; I had in fact already spent it on the television as I had assumed that the oversight would not be discovered. My denial was accepted on trust, and no further questions were asked. However, it was dishonest and when setting out moral frames the question always arises of how far the practice of espousing a moral intuition such as Honesty corresponds with the advocate's own practice. But I suppose I

© The Author(s), under exclusive license to Springer Nature Switzerland AG 2021
J. Charteris-Black, *Metaphors of Coronavirus*,
https://doi.org/10.1007/978-3-030-85106-4_10

was working on the principle that the error on this occasion to my benefit was a rare event. It is surely much more common to experience an unexpected charge, a tax one didn't know about, or to be a victim of fraud, so at times our moral intuitions about Fairness do not sit easily with those for Honesty: in this case, so I managed to convince myself, I was balancing the scales of justice because at other times I had been the victim of dishonesty, and I have some quite long tales to narrate about that too. In terms of Haidt's metaphor introduced in chapter one, surely this was a case of the rampant elephant of intuition overriding the rider of reason.

I have illustrated in this book how metaphor was essential to the moral framing of the pandemic whether at the level of particular metaphor frames, such as the 'war' or 'force of nature' frames or at the more allegorical level in terms of a zombie apocalypse or the 'we are the virus' allegory that proposed that the Coronavirus pandemic was Nature's retribution on humanity because of mankind's destructive impact on the environment. I have demonstrated how various moral intuitions such as Fairness and Cheating, and Sanctity and Degradation were aroused by the metaphors that were chosen by politicians and policy makers such as 'bubbles' and 'cocoons' and metonyms such as the 'China virus' and visual metonyms such as mask-wearing. I have also illustrated how opponents of government policy equally relied on metaphors such as 'petri dish' or on allegories based on the human body. I have proposed that the pandemic caused a fundamental change in moral intuitions away from exclusive reliance on 'the elephant' of emotional intuition towards 'the rider' of reason, truth, and the moral intuition of Honesty. This is because the basic principles of truth seeking that underlie medical scientific research into disease and its causes and the development of a vaccine need to dispel metaphors that contribute to a lack of trust in medical researchers or the vaccinations they propose, to expiate the false arguments of those who argue that Lockdown was just about scaring the population into submission or the vaccine was part of a global plot. Only by searching for a common moral framework based on empirical research and trust in public medicine can human survival be made a more feasible endeavor.

Although the war frame—with its metaphors of 'weapons' and 'front-line' staff—had its critics, especially for those without direct experience of war—framing the response as a strategic conflict between two sides—humanity and the virus—was well motivated because there is a basis in biological reality for this framing. Such 'war' metaphors had a significant influence on people's evaluation of various responses such as observing quarantine and presumably on their own behaviour (even if they were not always aware of this). We should recall that Susan Sontag in her *Metaphors of Illness* was not opposed to the war frame for its own sake but because of the damaging effect it could have on the lived experience of patients suffering from cancer (and later AIDS): if terms such as 'invasive' were used, they could feel as if defeat was a result of personal failings and the lack of resolution to fight. The reliance on the war frame in the initial phase of Covid-19 was because of the absence of another readily available frame for a disaster caused by two competing entities and it communicated the need for an urgent and robust social response to the threat posed by Covid-19—a threat that had been aggravated by an initially weak governmental response. Although few had direct experience of war, the frame itself had been kept alive through cultural history: commemorative events at airfields, interviews with war veterans, school projects on family history and of course the reporting of sports events that were invariably constructed in the discourse of war. So, while there may not have been the lived experience of war, there was an *imagined* experience of war.

Similarly, there was, in Europe (including the UK) and in the Americas, a complete absence of either lived or imagined experience of a pandemic. There had of course been SARS, MERS, Zika and Ebola but these had all been at a considerable geographical distance, in Asia or Africa. Epidemics in the UK such as foot and mouth disease or mad cow disease affected animals rather than humans. Parts of the world where there was a far greater degree of preparedness, and therefore less need for a war frame, arose from the lived experience of pandemics. Bearing in mind these reservations, in the British context, the war frame offered a source of comfort for many because it offered a familiar frame for a highly unfamiliar situation and in doing so was reassuring, here we were again: on the 'frontline'. However, metaphors such as the 'Blitz spirit' were shown empirically to be unappealing, especially to younger audiences, as they were now outmoded and did not reflect contemporary experience.

'Fire' metaphors were effective in explaining the rapidity with which the virus spread, how it could be stopped and provided moral commentary on how government policies could deliberately encourage the spread of the virus by 'adding fuel to the fire', 'fanning its flames' or 'pouring petrol on the flames'. As with 'war' metaphors, they alerted people to the urgency of the crisis and therefore aroused the moral intuition of Care and Harm. Similarly, 'force of nature' metaphors—such as 'overwhelmed', 'battered', 'waves' of coronavirus and 'surge' testing—contributed to a heightening the sense of crisis by arousing emotions and therefore invoked a social response. Metaphors such as 'turning the tide' on the virus also motivated people by providing a sense of the potential for concerted effort and the possibility of overcoming the virus. We have also heard how sufferers of Covid-19 often mixed their metaphors when expressing the emotional experience of their health crisis in a chaos narrative.

As well as such well-motivated metaphors that encouraged social cohesion, I have also argued that metaphors were important in politicians' accounts of the epidemiology of Covid-19 because they offered moral justification for their own policies. An electorate that had consistently been persuaded through its emotions, especially during the Brexit campaign when Loyalty and Betrayal had been a dominant moral intuition, was now asked by government to behave based on the moral intuitions of Care and Harm and Fairness and Cheating. The rider was getting back in control of the elephant. However, government was not trusted as its own performance did not always correspond with its claims. Metaphors such as 'following the science' and being 'led by the science' hardly matched with the lax initial response to the virus and the privileging of economic considerations over epidemiological ones or with the behaviour of some working for the government. They were overused and were later replaced by 'data not dates' in discussing the schedule for the re-opening of post-Lockdown society. Some concepts such as 'herd immunity' were improperly understood by commentators as they were treated as metaphors whereas in reality 'herd immunity' is a literal term for a scientific concept whereby a population gains immunity, irrespective of whether this is achieved by the natural response of the human immune system or by vaccination. As many as 39% of people could not properly explain it and probably distrusted it so further demonstrating how the moral intuition of Honesty and Dishonesty influenced both trust in government and public understanding of science. However, those who dreamt that the pandemic response measures were a cure that was worse than the disease seemed to be riding the elephant of Lockdown denial and vaccine hesitancy.

A number of metaphors based on the visual shape of graphs such as 'spikes', 'flattening the curve' and 'squashing the sombrero' appealed to the moral intuition of Care and Harm but were perhaps too descriptive to be of great effect in influencing actions. By contrast, newer metaphors such as 'circuit breaker' were more effective in combining the dual goals of intelligibility and influencing behaviour by advocating actions with which most people concurred. In terms of their accessibility to the public, metaphor-based scientific concepts were often better understood than literal, technical terms. For example, around 78% of people could explain three of the metaphor-based terms discussed in Chap. 5. What characterized a metaphor such as 'circuit breaker' is that, in addition to communicating a science-based concept, it displaced agency from the government to scientific experts. By drawing on scientific metaphors, public policy was attributed to the agency of scientists and epidemiologists who were more trusted than politicians. This demonstrates that how the moral intuition of Honesty and Dishonesty could be influenced by the language used in the public communication of politicians. It also leads us to expect that they will themselves follow the rules and laws they have created—something that was evidently not the case with either Dominic Cummings, or, once he had been dismissed, his major target: Matt Hancock who, rather unexpectedly, turned out to be something of a Romeo.

Confinement is an embodied experience that has, throughout history, motivated metaphors and metonyms during pandemics and provided a frame of containment that became the basis for understanding the relationship between the individual's *body*, and, through language, *the body politic* or society. This becomes greatly accentuated in times of pandemic because there is a medical need to confine humans to particular locations: confinement is necessary for social survival. The infected body is placed within a designated structure: a house, a hospital, an intensive care unit and the possibly infected body is confined within actual or notional boundaries that impose limits on its movement. Medical professionals are confined to hazmat suits, and everyone is told to 'stay at home and save lives'. Confinement is an embodied experience that can either be imposed by external forces or selected by the individual and in Chap. 6 we saw evidence of both these practices in Defoe's account of the plague. I then explored how confinement as embodied experience contributed to a container frame through specific metaphors that characterized public discussion of the coronavirus pandemic. I identified a contrast between containers such as 'bubbles', 'cocoons', 'pods' and 'protective rings' that attribute value to what is contained and those such as 'pockets' and 'silos' that place negative value on what is inside the container. I also pointed out the covert moral coercion implied by the 'cocoon' metaphor and the lack of substance in the 'bubbles' metaphor, as well as their tendency to 'burst'. The 'petri dish' was a rather different metaphor as it placed a negative evaluation of the intentions and purposes of the agent that put the entity into the container rather than what is contained within. What these metaphors share is their diverse appeal to a wide range of moral intuitions including Care and Harm, Loyalty and Betrayal, Fairness and Cheating, Sanctity and Degradation—and as I have argued throughout this book, Honesty and Dishonesty. When government advisers develop seductive metaphors to enforce policies that they then do not then themselves adhere to it shakes the moral foundations so that the house of government could collapse.

At the allegorical level the Zombie Apocalypse frame and 'We are the virus' meme both drew on fantasy and science fiction to express moral emotions. Both expressed feelings of a loss of agency and both were somewhat fatalistic in the face of the powerful forces of nature that had been unleashed by coronavirus. People could lose their powers of reason and become slaves of the zombie virus and so were not only carriers of the virus but also *became the virus itself.* Both the 'Zombie' frame and 'We are the virus' memes, and others too from Science Fiction, put humanity in a vulnerable position and to the extent that we were all in it together—whether against a zombie outbreak or a pandemic—they appealed to the elephant of intuition. Another similarity is that both memes carried with them the gratification of an 'I told you so' sentiment—followers of the zombie genre were, it seems, well prepared psychologically for the pandemic, because the empty streets and enforced reduction of social contract confirmed their views that there had *always* been a danger of the zombie outbreak.

'We are the virus' allegories confirmed the intuitions of those concerned about man's impact on the environment and showed the true extent of pollution and how this impacted negatively on nature, so validating pre-existing fears and anxieties. Both Science Fiction frames also had important similarities in terms of their emergent space, the Zombie Apocalypse frame included an allegory that just as the virus mutated to avoid detection, so humanity could evolve to develop protection against zombies, indeed the pandemic provided the perfect scenario for testing how far social mechanisms could survive a zombie outbreak by adaptation to it. The 'We are the virus' frame had in its emergent space an allegory that if we are the virus, then we can develop vaccines against the virus; if the vaccine offers protection against the virus of humanity, then zero carbon emissions, and other policies that prioritise nature can be the vaccine that saves humanity from destroying our environment. But these emergent spaces of Science Fiction are based on restoring reason as the rider over intuitions. One final similarity is that, as internet memes, both also offered the potential for creative elaboration from multiple authors through the processes of parody and comment. Individuals everywhere could creatively reimagine the pandemic in such a way that allowed humour, fantasy, and expression of moral emotions in contested and complementary allegories, and this was in fact an honest response to challenge the annoying certainty of those who always thought they knew how it would all pan out in terms of species survival.

However, as well as these structural parallels, the two frames pulled in rather different directions in terms of the moral psychology of their allegories: the 'We are the virus' meme, until it was parodied, offered a condemnation of humanity and its impact on nature: based on the moral intuition of Degradation it took the side of nature against mankind. Conversely the 'Zombie' allegory did not argue that it would be morally right for zombies to take over the planet and destroy humanity, it encouraged the type of unified and planned rational response in defence of humanity against this viral outbreak of nature and so appealed more to the moral intuitions of Care and Harm and of Loyalty (to the human species)—as well as to reason. And the fact that the zombies were a relatively slow-moving and soft target offered the prospect that as part of this allegory victory was possible—such optimism was perhaps lacking among many proponents of the 'We are the virus' meme, though more present in those parodying it. The truth is that if you know it's a zombie you will either avoid it or take it out.

We have also explored the role of metaphors such as 'silver bullet' and 'magic wand' in making arguments both in favour of a vaccine for Covid-19 and in warnings against over-expectations regarding such vaccines, and traced these back to theories such as The Magic Bullet Theory of the power of mass media. We found that 'magic bullets' and 'silver bullets' are often expressed in negative forms—'no magic/ silver bullet' and are intended to frame opposing positions as childish and Dishonest and so perform expectation management. Mixed in with the magic we have Hancock's dishonest 'protective ring' around the care homes—dishonest because many elderly people suffering from Covid-19 were forced from hospitals into care homes without being tested. I have shown that the expression 'miracle cure' was used ironically in the press as a means of exposing the numerous fake remedies proposed for Covid-19 and therefore also appealed to the moral intuition of Honesty and Dishonesty.

I have illustrated how vaccine discourse—when arguing for and against a Covid-19 vaccination—relies on metaphors that arouse moral intuitions. I have shown how, historically, metaphoric thinking in the anti-vaccine movement blends the human with the animal by associating vaccination with contamination and degradation of the body and spirit and appeals to the moral intuition of Sanctity and Degradation. It's a view on the world that appeals entirely to the emotional intuition of the elephant. People adopt mental models about vaccine from early influences, for example their family, or religious or political leaders, people whom they judge to be honest. These are often based on whether they themselves were vaccinated as children, their personal models for the human body and its relations to the animal body. They then search in echo chambers for whatever occurs in news reports, or the anecdotes of their social circle that confirms these moral intuitions. These pre-existing intuitions are exploited by propagandists when seeking to influence through metaphor. Equally, public scientists, politicians, journalists, and others seeking to expose information as deliberately misleading, also rely on metaphors such as 'miracle cure' when establishing their arguments; these are clearly appealing to the instinctive elephant.

In conclusion, the pandemic has offered a refocusing of Moral Foundations Theory by repositioning the rider back in control over the elephant, and suggests the argument that honesty can aid species survival. Nations with honest leaders who follow the rules they have created will survive longer than those with corrupt and dishonest leaders. A rampaging elephant, like a rampant virus, represents an immanent and present danger that requires control through reasoned response. If democratic leaders can regain trust, first through their own behavior, and then by providing policies that encourage mutual protection of the planet, and the species that at present occupy it, they can, as well as saving humanity, *give to species that do not yet exist the opportunity to do so*. If leaders of non-democracies can find a common purpose in these objectives, then they become still more attainable. Language has a crucial role to play in all this drama, not by rejecting metaphor and allegory, and not by deception and dishonesty, but by finding honest language, including metaphors, that corresponds with embodied experience, that reinforce reason, and enhances the life, health, and pleasure of humanity.

References

Ackerman, J., Tybur, J. M., & Blackwell, A. D. (2020). What role does pathogen avoidance pyschology play in pandemics? *Trends in Cognitive Sciences, 25*, 177–186.

Ariely, D. (2008). *Predicably irrational: The hidden forces that shape our decisions.* Harper Collins.

Biss, E. (2014). *On immunity.* Fitzcarraldo Editions.

Burnet, F. M., & Clark, E. (1942). *Influenza: A survey of the last fifty years* (Monograph from the Walter and Eliza Hall Institute of Research in Pathology and Medicine, no 4). Macmillan.

Camus, A. (1947). *La Peste.* R. Buss (Trans.). Penguin.

Charteris-Black, J. (2004). *Corpus approaches to critical metaphor analysis.* Palgrave Macmillan.

Charteris-Black, J. (2006). Britain as a container: Immigration metaphors in the 2005 election campaign. *Discourse & Society, 17*(6), 563–582.

Charteris-Black, J. (2012). Shattering the bell jar: Metaphor, gender and depression. *Metaphor & Symbol, 27*, 199–216.

Charteris-Black, J. (2016). The 'dull roar' and the 'burning barbed wire pantyhose; Complex metaphor in accounts of chronic pain. In R. W. Gibbs (Ed.), *Mixing metaphor* (pp. 155–178). Benjamins.

© The Author(s), under exclusive license to Springer Nature Switzerland AG 2021
J. Charteris-Black, *Metaphors of Coronavirus*,
https://doi.org/10.1007/978-3-030-85106-4

Charteris-Black, J. (2017a). *Fire metaphors: Discourses of awe and authority*. Bloomsbury.

Charteris-Black, J. (2017b). Competition metaphors & ideology: Life as a race. In R. Wodak & B. Forchtner (Eds.), *The Routledge handbook of language and politics* (pp. 202–217). Routledge.

Charteris-Black, J. (2018). *Analysing political speeches:Rrhetoric, discourse and metaphor* (2nd ed.). Palgrave Macmillan.

Charteris-Black, J. (2019). *Metaphors of Brexit: No cherries on the cake?* Palgrave Macmillan.

Chilton, P. (1996). *Security metaphors: Cold War discourse from containment to common house*. Peter Lang.

Chilton, P. (2004). *Analysing political discourse*. Routledge.

Chmara, T. (2015). Do minors have first amendment rights in schools? *Knowledge Quest, 44*(1), 8–13.

Dodsworth, L. (2021). *A state of fear: How the UK government weaponised fear during the Covid-19 pandemic*. Pinter & Martin.

Fauconnier, G., & Turner, M. (2002). *The way we think: Conceptual blending and the mind's hidden complexities*. Basic Books.

Feng, W. D. (2017). Metonymy and visual representation: Towards a social semiotic framework of visual metonymy. *Visual Communication, 16*(4), 441–466.

Flusberg, S. J., Matlock, T., & Thibodeau, P. H. (2018). War metaphors in public discourse. *Metaphor and Symbol, 33*(1), 1–18.

Forceville, C. (2009). Metonymy in visual and audiovisual discourse. In E. Ventola & A. J. M. Guijarro (Eds.), *The world told and the world shown: Issues in multisemiotics* (pp. 56–74). Palgrave Macmillan.

Frank, A. W. (1995). *The wounded storyteller: Body, illness, and ethics*. University of Chicago Press.

Gibbs, R. W. (1990). Psycholinguistic studies on the conceptual basis of idiomaticity. *Cognitive Linguistics, 1*, 417–451.

Gibbs, R. W. (1994). *The poetics of mind: Figurative thought, language, and understanding*. Cambridge University Press.

Gibbs, R. W. (Ed.). (2016). *Mixing metaphor*. John Benjamins.

Haidt, J. (2012). *The righteous mind*. Penguin.

Ho, J., & Chiang, E. (2021). 'Those lunatic zombies': The discursive framing of Wuhan lockdown escapees in digital space. In A. Musolff, R. Breeze, S. Vilar-Lluch, & K. Kondon (Eds.), *Pandemic and crisis discourse* (pp. 484–508). Bloomsbury.

Honigsbaum, M. (2020). *The pandemic century: A history of global contagion from the Spanish flu to Covid-19*. Allen.

Joffe, H., & Haarhoff, G. (2002). Representations of far-flung illnesses: The case of Ebola in Britain. *Social Science & Medicine, 54*(6), 955–969.

Khan, A. (2021). Identity as crime: How Indian mainstream media's coverage demonised Muslims as Coronavirus spreaders. In A. Musolff, R. Breeze, S. Vilar-Lluch, & K. Kondon (Eds.), *Pandemic and crisis discourse* (pp. 514–538). Bloomsbury.

Kövecses, Z. (2003). *Metaphor and emotion: Language, culture and body in human feeling.* CUP.

Kövecses, Z. (2010). *Metaphor: A practical introduction.* Oxford University Press.

Lakoff, G. (1991). The metaphor system used to justify war in the gulf. *Journal of Urban and Cultural Studies, 2*(1), 59–72.

Lakoff, G., & Johnson, M. (1980). *Metaphors we live by.* University of Chicago Press.

Lakoff, G., & Turner, M. (1989). *More than cool reason: A field guide to poetic metaphor.* University of Chicago Press.

Larson, B. M., Nerlich, B., & Wallis, P. (2005). Metaphors and biorisks: The war on infectious diseases and invasive species. *Science Communication, 26*(3), 243–268.

Levinovitz, A. (2020). *Natural: How faith in nature's goodness leads to harmful fads, unjust laws and flawed science.* Beacon Press.

Louw, B. (1993). Irony in the text or insincerity in the writer?—The diagnostic potential of semantic prosodies. In M. Baker, G. Francis, & E. Tognini-Bonelli (Eds.), *Text & technology: In honour of John Sinclair* (pp. 157–176). Benjamins.

Masters-Waage, T. C., Jha, N., & Reb, J. (2020). COVID-19, Coronavirus, Wuhan virus, or China virus? Understanding how to "do no harm" when naming an infectious disease. *Frontiers in Psychology, 11*, 561270.

Musolff, A. (2021). "War against COVID-19": Is the pandemic as war metaphor helpful or hurtful? In A. Musolff, R. Breeze, S. Vilar-Lluch, & K. Kondo (Eds.), *Pandemic and crisis discourse: Communicating COVID-19 and public health strategy.* Bloomsbury.

Nerlich, B. (2020). Metaphors in times of coronavirus. Retrieved June 18, 2021, from https://blogs.nottingham.ac.uk/makingsciencepublic/2020/03/17/metaphors-in-the-time-of-coronavirus/

Nerlich, B., & Jaspal, R. (2021). Social representations of 'social distancing' in response to Covid-19 in the UK media. *Current Sociology, 69*(4), 1–18. https://doi.org/10.1177/0011392121990030

Nerlich, H., & Halliday, C. (2007). Avian flu: The creation of expectations in the interplay between science and the media. *Sociology of Health and Illness, 29*(1), 46–65.

Oborne, P. (2012). *The assault on truth: Boris Johnson, Donald Trump and the emergence of a new moral barbarism*. Simon & Schuster.

Oswick, C., Grant, D., & Oswick, R. (2020). Categories, crossroads, control, connectedness, continuity, and change: A metaphorical exploration of COVID-19. *Journal of Applied Behavioural Science, 56*(3), 284–288.

Semino, E. (2021). "Not soldiers but fire-fighters"—Metaphors and Covid-19. *Health Communication, 36*(1), 50–58.

Silaški, N., & Đurović, T. (2021). From an invisible enemy to a football match with the virus: Adjusting the COVID-19 pandemic metaphors to political agendas in Serbian public discourse. In A. Musolff, R. Breeze, S. Vilar-Lluch, & K. Kondo (Eds.), *Pandemic and crisis discourse: Communicating COVID-19 and Public health strategy*. Bloomsbury.

Sontag, S. (1989). *Illness as metaphor and AIDS and its metaphors*. Penguin Modern Classics.

Talmy, L. (1988). Force dynamics in language and cognition. *Cognitive Science, 12*(1), 49–100.

Thibodeau, P. H., & Boroditsky, L. (2011). Metaphors we think with: The role of metaphor in reasoning. *PloS ONE, 6*(2), e16782.

Thomas, K. (1991). *Religion and the decline of magic*. Penguin.

Wallis, P., & Nerlich, B. (2005). Disease metaphors in new epidemics: The UK media framing of the 2003 SARS epidemic. *Social Science & Medicine, 60*, 2629–2639.

White, C. F. (1935). Plague: Modern preventive measures in ships and ports. *Proceedings of the Royal Society of Medicine, 28*(5), 591–602.

Wolfe, R. M., & Sharpe, L. K. (2002). Anti-vaccinationists past and present. *BMJ, 325*, 430–432.

Yu, Y. (2021). Legitimising a global fight for a shared future: A critical metaphor analysis of the reportage of COVID-19 in *China Daily*. In A. Musolff, R. Breeze, S. Vilar-Lluch, & K. Kondo (Eds.), *Pandemic and crisis discourse: Communicating COVID-19 and public health strategy*. Bloomsbury. Chapter 14.

Index[1]

---

[1] Note: Page numbers followed by 'n' refer to notes.

© The Author(s), under exclusive license to Springer Nature Switzerland AG 2021
J. Charteris-Black, *Metaphors of Coronavirus*,
https://doi.org/10.1007/978-3-030-85106-4